Social Work and Mental Health

Social Work in Theory and Practice series

Kate Karban, *Social Work and Mental Health*
Ann McDonald, *Social Work with Older People*
Roger Smith, *Social Work with Young People*

Skills for Contemporary Social Work series

Tony Evans & Mark Hardy, *Evidence and Knowledge for Practice*
Andrew Hill, *Working in Statutory Contexts*

Social Work and Mental Health

KATE KARBAN

polity

First published in 2011 by Polity Press

Polity Press
65 Bridge Street
Cambridge CB2 1UR, UK

Polity Press
350 Main Street
Malden, MA 02148, USA

ISBN-13: 978-0-7456-4610-7
ISBN-13: 978-0-7456-4611-4(pb)

A catalogue record for this book is available from the
British Library.

Typeset in 9.5 on 12 pt Utopia
by Toppan Best-set Premedia Limited

The publisher has used its best endeavours to ensure that
the URLs for external websites referred to in this book are
correct and active at the time of going to press. However,
the publisher has no responsibility for the websites and
can make no guarantee that a site will remain live or that
the content is or will remain appropriate.

Every effort has been made to trace all copyright holders,
but if any have been inadvertently overlooked the publisher will be pleased to include any necessary credits in
any subsequent reprint or edition.

For further information on Polity, visit our website: www.
politybooks.com

Contents

Acknowledgements

Thanks are due to the many students and colleagues at Leeds Metropolitan University and the University of Bradford. Too numerous to name, they have helped to shape and influence this book. Particular thanks are due to friends and family who have offered encouragement as well as valuable insights and knowledge. The book would not have been completed without Hazel's support and constructive comments, and, as always, Laura and Alex continue to inspire me with their enthusiasm and creativity.

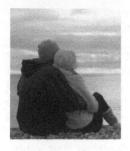

Introduction

Key points

- Definition of mental health
- Mental health as a global concern
- The contribution of social work to mental health
- Developing a critical and reflective response to mental health in social work practice

Issues and Themes

This introduction will highlight the key issues that will be developed through the book, beginning by locating mental health in a wider national and global context as a major public health concern. Some initial discussion on the meaning of terms and use of language as well as some basic facts and figures will also be presented. The relationship between mental health and issues of inequality and disadvantage will be introduced, indicating where these issues will be developed further.

The range and scope of the role of social work in responding to mental health issues will be outlined, linked to the rationale for the approach of this book, which is that mental health is a key element of all areas of social work practice. The particular contribution that social work has made to mental health thinking and practice will be recognized and areas of future development will also be highlighted.

Finally, some of the challenges offered by the development of integrated services, interprofessional working and working in partnership with service users and carers will be raised, offering a critical approach to practice and recognizing the complexities of the current emphasis on evidence-based practice.

Who Might Find This Book of Interest?

This book is intended to be of relevance to anyone interested in social work, whether or not they are students or practitioners, and regardless of setting. It is recognized, however, that the main audience is likely to be social work students working towards qualification on either undergraduate or postgraduate courses, as well as qualified practitioners who want to update their knowledge of mental health or who are engaged in post-qualifying training or other forms of continuing professional development. In particular the book is designed to challenge the idea that it is only social workers in specialist mental health teams who 'do' mental health work. Instead, the view that all social workers are engaged in the business of promoting mental health and wellbeing will be emphasized, recognizing that some may have a particular role in working with people experiencing longer-term and more serious mental health difficulties.

With the continuing emphasis on interprofessional and multi-agency working, it is also anticipated that the book may be of interest to others working in mental health or in related health and social care settings. With increasing attention being paid to mental health issues in the wider community and across other sectors, and growing interest in social perspectives and the impact of social inequalities, others such as community support workers, assistant and associate practitioners, as well as nurses and occupational therapists, may find particular chapters relevant.

'Mental Health is Everyone's Business'

This slogan emphasizes that mental health is a major global concern affecting all of us. Evidence from the World Health Organization (WHO) indicates that in 2004, over 150 million people worldwide experienced depression and 26 million people had a diagnosis of schizophrenia. Additionally, 40 million people suffered from epilepsy and 24 million from Alzheimer's disease and other dementias, and 125 million people were affected by alcohol use disorders (WHO, 2008). Nationally the figures are no less significant, with 8.65 million people in the UK experiencing mental health disorders in 2007, projected to rise to 9.88 million by 2026, accompanied by rising costs, including service costs and lost earnings, increasing from £48.6 billion to £60.69 billion by 2026 (McCrone et al., 2008).

Whilst it is beyond the scope of this book to extend to a comprehensive global perspective, it will, on occasions, be important to recognize the cross-cutting links and connections with mental health issues and practice in other parts of the world, acknowledging wider international trends and the need to be open to learning from others, sometimes in very different circumstances. From the Alma-Ata declaration in 1978 to the Millennium Development Goals, the values of social justice and equity transcend both international and organizational boundaries between health and social care, highlighting the wider costs and risk factors associated with long-term health conditions (Chan, 2008). This message has also been reinforced by the Report of the Commission on the Social Determinants of Health (2008), which draws attention to the need for health care systems to respond to underlying social, economic and political causes of ill health. More specifically, with respect to mental health, there is an increasing recognition that there is 'no health without mental health' (WHO, 2005: 11) and that there is a two-way relationship between mental disorders and other health conditions, with mental health difficulties increasing the risk for other health conditions, and the presence of physical ill health increasing the chance of mental illness. Furthermore, health services are not available or accessible on an equitable basis for people experiencing mental health problems, increasing the risk of further health difficulties (Prince et al., 2007).

Mental Health, Human Rights and Social Justice

Mental health, as one element of health in general, is also an issue of human rights and social justice, as asserted in the following statement from the International Federation of Social Workers (IFSW): 'These two central social work values frame IFSW's understanding that all people have an equal right to enjoy the social conditions that underpin human health and to access services and other resources to promote health and deal with illness' (International Federation of Social Workers, 2008).

It is no coincidence that the greatest challenges to promoting and supporting mental wellbeing concern inequality, disadvantage and discrimination. Notions of social justice will be central in exploring both theory and practice, requiring the critical appraisal of evidence from a variety of sources and a reflective approach to the material presented.

In this sense mental health can be seen to be at the heart of social work, defined as 'a profession which promotes social change, problem solving in human relationships and the empowerment and liberation of people to enhance well-being. Utilising theories of human behaviour and social systems, social work intervenes at the points where people interact with their environments. Principles of human rights and social justice are fundamental to social work' (International Association of Schools of Social Work/International Federation of Social Workers, 2001).

Social Work and Mental Health

An important message that this book hopes to convey is that social work has a vital contribution to make to mental health, drawing on the values, knowledge and skills of the profession. The message is especially significant when moves towards the integration of services across health and social care are sometimes experienced by social workers as leaving them in a twilight zone where they feel marginalized and undervalued. The historical development of social work as a profession, looking back to the early twentieth century, includes the first training course at the London School of Economics, the recommendations of the 1939 Feversham Report for minimum standards and training for mental health social workers and the 1959 Younghusband Report referring to the need for training and employment of psychiatric social workers (Timms, 1964). Developments in anti-discriminatory and anti-oppressive practice of the 1980s and 1990s were also accompanied by changes in the statutory and legislative role of social workers in mental health. These and other factors have all been influential in shaping the current situation and the potential future role that social work has to play in mental health.

Although this text is not organized on the basis of a lifespan approach to mental health, addressing each discrete stage from childhood through to old age, many aspects of mental health through the lifespan will be addressed in the various chapters. Again the message is that not only are all social workers engaged in mental health work, but they are embedded within a complex web of relationships with other professionals and agencies, as well as with families, carers and individuals.

As with other professions, social work is facing the challenges associated with professional regulation and registration. Some of the issues associated with this will be explored further, acknowledging both the opportunities and the threats inherent in such developments. In particular it is important to recognize the tensions and contradictions caused by what can be understood as a move towards deprofessionalization on the one hand and the need for an increasingly skilled and knowledgeable workforce within a world of finite economic and financial resources on the other.

With regard to mental health this can be found in the New Working Ways (Care Sector Improvement Partnership/National Institute for Mental Health in England, 2007) agenda, highlighting the need for flexible roles across multiprofessional teams, with an emphasis on particular skills rather than specific professions. This can be seen in the replacement of the Approved Social Worker with the Approved Mental Health Professional role, open to suitably qualified nurses, occupational therapists and psychologists as well as social workers, as part of the Mental Health Act 2007, which also offers opportunities for social workers and other professions to take on the new role of Responsible Clinician.

There are also increasing numbers of professionally non-aligned workers, including health or social care assistants, many of whom have first-hand experience of mental health difficulties. Undertaking valuable work in housing support, social inclusion and recovery, their role also raises important questions about what is the contribution of social work. At the same time there is a need to ensure that people in such roles have access to opportunities for further training and qualifications.

Of central importance is the integration of the professional role with the expectations of service users and carers and the underpinning values of social work.

> Social work does bring something distinctive to the mental health arena . . . It is a constellation of values, commitment to social justice,

> partnership with users and carers, the ability to see the social context of individuals and how this influences both behaviours and recovery, and a commitment to the worth of each individual which meant social workers practiced social inclusion before the term had been invented. Above all it stands as a challenge to the traditional medical model of diagnosis, prescription and treatment which does not fully acknowledge the mental health service user as best informed about their needs. (Social Perspectives Network, n.d.)

Duggan points to the following four reasons for articulating the social model which is seen to be pivotal to the social work contribution to mental health:

- the policy emphasis on partnership and collaboration
- developments in service user and citizen involvement
- the multi-factorial nature of the new public health agenda
- evidence for the effectiveness of holistic interventions aimed at the root causes of ill health and health inequality.

(Duggan et al., 2002: 5)

In turn, these reasons inform the debate that will unfold thorough the chapters of this text, contributing to the creation of a flexible framework for social work practice and underpinned by a clear value base.

A Word on Language

Throughout this book you will encounter a range of terminology to describe mental health difficulties. The underpinning conceptual issues will be explored in a later chapter but it is important to note here the variety of language that will be used, with terms such as 'mental health problems', 'mental health difficulties' and 'mental ill health' being used interchangeably. Most importantly, terms that label an individual in the diagnosis, such as a schizophrenic, will be avoided. The terms used will reflect language that is currently used and accepted by people who have lived experience of such difficulties, recognizing that there is no overall consensus or agreement.

Where appropriate, the term 'service user' will be used where it relates specifically to the experience of using services, recognizing that many people experiencing mental health problems choose not to access or do not have access to mental health services. The term 'survivor' may also be used where appropriate. The term 'carers' will be used to describe those who provide care informally, often family members, friends or neighbours. References to carers who are employed in a formal capacity will make this clear.

In places, terms that would be deemed unacceptable in current terminology will be used within their historical context, reflecting previous common usage, such as 'lunatics', 'mental handicap' or 'mental defective'. This should be clear to the reader, but where necessary, these terms will be used in quotes to indicate their historical nature.

Reflective Practice

Reflective practice will be a continuing theme which will inform the analysis and discussion throughout this book, and will underpin the discussion points and questions that will be contained within each chapter. Inherent within this will be a model of critical reflection that will promote in-depth thinking and questioning, an essential requirement both for achieving qualifying, post-qualifying and academic awards, and for making sense of the complexity of practice and developing ways of responding to the challenges of new and changing situations.

The approach to reflective practice here has drawn on the work of Fook (2002), who has challenged modernist ways of thinking about knowledge and practice. In its place she proposes that a postmodern perspective is necessary to draw attention to 'the diverse number of ways in which we can understand and make knowledge, and therefore the many different types and theories of practices which exist, and the many different ways in which they relate to each other' (2002: 44). This is relevant to the approach taken in this text in attempting to offer a broad approach to social work and mental health. The range of social work settings and areas of practice coupled with the complexities of interprofessional and multi-agency working, particularly with health colleagues, has inevitably meant that at points, there may be tensions and conflicts. An example of this concerns the discussion about psychosocial intervention when working with people experiencing psychosis, where the evidence-based nature of this approach may seem to be at odds with the more constructivist stance advocated elsewhere. As in the realities of day-to-day practice, there is a need to avoid simplistic binary thinking based on two opposing positions. Instead, it is sometimes necessary to look for common ground, in the process contributing to the continuing debate and exploration which move theory and practice forward and increase our understanding.

The Structure of the Book

Inevitably, when putting together a text of this kind, there are difficult decisions to be made. These include not only what to leave out and what to keep in, but also how to organize the content in a way that makes sense to the reader, offering both coherence and the development of certain key themes that recur throughout. The structure of this book therefore contains certain compromises and tensions, in part reflecting the complex and multifaceted nature of the subject.

As an example, whilst there is no chapter dedicated to the carers of people with mental health difficulties, these issues are addressed in a number of relevant chapters, including Chapter 1 on the experiences of users and carers and Chapters 3 and 4 on policy and legislation, as well as being integrated into the chapters on practice where appropriate.

Overall the book is organized in three main parts. Part 1 provides an introduction to some of the key perspectives on mental health, including that of services users and others who have experienced mental distress, various models for understanding mental health, and a policy/legal perspective. Part 2 moves on to consider key aspects of the evidence base underpinning social perspectives in mental health which are seen as essential elements of the social work knowledge base in this area. Part 3 offers a number of practice-focused chapters, addressing social work in both mental health and other settings.

Chapter 1 begins with the voices of people who have themselves experienced mental distress and who may have received mental health services, recognizing a long tradition of survival and resistance both nationally and internationally. Reference will be made to the historical origins and continuing impact and influence of the user movement as well as to the experiences of carers. Chapter 2 offers an introduction to the medical model and other ways of understanding mental health and illness, which themselves inform and underpin various approaches to the delivery of mental health services. Issues of current policy form the content of Chapter 3, which also traces the historical development of key policy themes and relates current issues to social work practice. Chapter 4 addresses the legal context for mental health social work, drawing on a range of relevant legislation, including the Mental Health Act 2007 and the Mental Capacity Act 2005. It is important to note that whilst reference will be made to the current legislation in Scotland and Northern Ireland, it is beyond the scope of this text to address this in detail, and the main emphasis will be on the law and policy pertaining to England and Wales.

Part 2 comprises two chapters which together provide core evidence for the central importance of a social perspective. Chapter 5 begins with a discussion on the social determinants of health and the challenge these pose for a traditional, individualistic and largely medical model, and moves on to consider the relevance of concepts of community and social capital for mental health. This leads into Chapter 6, which highlights particular aspects of diversity and oppression that characterize the mental health experiences of certain groups and their access to services, in particular considering the mental health of Black and minority ethnic groups, the lesbian, gay and bisexual communities and issues of gender, recognizing the growing interest in and recognition of men's mental health as well as long-standing concerns about the mental health of women.

Issues of social work are brought to the fore in Part 3 with a series of chapters focusing on different aspects of practice. The first two chapters address lifespan issues, considering the opportunities to address mental health issues when working with, first, children and families (Chapter 7) and, second, older people (Chapter 8). Chapter 9 moves into the area of practice with people experiencing what are frequently described as common mental health problems, including depression and anxiety, paying attention to the increasing use of cognitive behavioural therapy in responding to such difficulties as well as to issues of trauma and abuse. The contribution of social work to working with people with psychosis is the main theme of Chapter 10, drawing on practice examples to demonstrate various aspects of collaborative working with an emphasis on engagement and working to promote recovery. The final chapter in Part 3 consider the challenges and tensions offered by the need to respond to issues of risk related to mental health, recognizing the need to balance the attention paid to risk and dangerousness with positive risk-taking and concern with wider risks such as those of social exclusion or loss of liberty. This chapter also foregrounds the importance of working with interprofessional and multi-agency networks and settings, and the need for effective communication and co-ordination between all the relevant practitioners involved in any one situation. Additionally, this chapter highlights some of the issues associated with working with someone with a diagnosis of personality disorder, although it is recognized that this diagnosis is itself controversial. Other aspects of personality disorder are addressed in Chapter 2 as well as Chapter 9, acknowledging the range of experiences and responses associated with this rather broad label.

Finally, the concluding chapter draws together the key themes of the book and identifies some of the issues that may influence and impact upon mental health social work in the future.

A number of vignettes from practice will be introduced to illustrate particular themes and issues and are intended to ensure that the experiences of individuals and their families remain at the heart of the book. Whilst drawn from the author's experience, these are not based on specific individuals. Each chapter will begin with a list of key points to guide the reader and will end with a brief conclusion to emphasize the issues that have been covered. Suggestions for further reading are also offered.

Taking Care of Our Own Mental Health

In reading this book and considering mental health and its relevance to social work, it is important to heed a health warning. Any one of us may experience mental health difficulties and indeed it is important to recognize that some readers of this text will themselves have such experiences. There is no clear-cut line between those who find themselves affected by poor mental health and those who do not, and at various points notions of 'them and us' will be challenged in the text.

In addition to the possibility that the stresses and strains of complex personal and professional lives may impact on our wellbeing, working with people who may be upset or in distress, who have experienced trauma or who are overwhelmed with bewildering experiences may also take its toll. Recognizing this risk is all the more pertinent given that a message for practice that runs through this book is the importance of building relationships with those who use services. Keeping (2008: 73) refers to the demands of 'emotional engagement', without which service users can become depersonalized and the work can develop a practical and administrative focus, emphasizing 'doing' rather than 'being'. Emotional engagement, however, requires that social workers are themselves provided with support in order for their own personal and sometimes difficult emotional responses to be understood. Without such support, ideally available through supervision, helpful and effective social work relationships may be difficult to achieve. Looking after our own wellbeing as social workers is therefore essential for the quality of all our relationships, both professional and personal.

PART 1

PERSPECTIVES ON MENTAL HEALTH

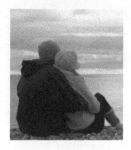

1 Voices from the Front Line: Users and Carers

Key points

- The experiences and perspectives of people with mental health difficulties
- Different approaches and responses to mental health issues
- The development of the service user 'movement'
- The concept of recovery and its impact on mental health
- The role and contribution of carers, recognizing shared and diverse interests

Introduction

This first chapter is intended to set the scene for the chapters that follow by focusing on the voices of those people who have experienced mental distress. The role and contribution of carers will also be explored. The chapter will begin by considering the experiences of service users in the past and will also refer to some of the literature associated with these experiences. We will then move on to consider the service user 'movement' and the development of user involvement in the later twentieth century, recognizing the influence of and tensions created by the rise of 'identity politics' as well as the influence of concepts of consumerism and citizenship. The statutory requirements for involvement and the different and sometimes contested priorities within the overall user involvement agenda will be considered before moving on to consider the concept of 'recovery' and its impact on the relationship between service users and services. Finally some of the issues associated with the role of carers will be introduced.

When reading this chapter and those that follow, it is also important to reflect on the issues of language and meaning in terms of the terminology that is used.

Reflection point

List as many different words as you can think of that may be used to describe people who use or potentially could use mental health services Then in relation to each word, think about what this term might convey to:
- someone who is described by this term;
- others who hear this language.

Some of the words that might be likely to be on your list are:

Patient
Service user
Client
Consumer
Customer
Survivor

This list excludes some of the terms that may have been used historically, such as 'inmate'. Each of these terms carries within it a suggestion of the kind of relationship that might be involved between the individual and the service. For example, the notion of being a 'patient' can suggest a passive recipient of care and treatment provided by professionals and experts who 'know best'. The terms 'consumer' and 'customer' indicate a relationship based on choice and rights within a marketplace where there are opportunities to pick and choose a service and also the right to decline a service altogether. Such opportunities are of course limited with respect to mental health care, where the choice as to whether or not to engage with services or the availability of a range of options is frequently not on offer. The term 'service user' is often used to denote a more neutral relationship whilst having the potential to obscure more complex power dynamics between the service and the recipient. However, many people have also rejected this term as having negative connotations associated with other 'users' of drugs. The concept of 'survivor' may be employed in relation to surviving either the mental distress itself or the services that have been available, and is a term preferred by some, but not all, people who have used or potentially could use services.

It would appear that there are no easy answers as to the most appropriate language to use. However, this brief discussion of terminology can remind us to consider our choice of language with care and to take every opportunity in practice to check out the preferences of individuals and to respect these in our own communication. In developing critical and reflective social work practice it will also be important to listen closely to the language that is used by other professionals as well as users and carers, and to consider the meanings that may be embedded within this. As Deegan (1996: 7) points out, changing language may obscure the continuation of relationships and services that perpetuate dependence and inequality.

An important message to be taken from this chapter is the need to avoid the 'othering' that can take place between professionals and people experiencing mental distress. This refers to the process by which professionals draw a line between 'us' and 'them' in a way that emphasizes, either implicitly or explicitly, the difference between the two. Such a process also contributes to the maintenance of exclusion or segregation: this may operate on a physical basis, such as that found in the old asylums, but can also exist in the continuation of practices and systems that emphasize 'them' and 'us' in the community.

To return to the use of the term 'patient': this can be seen as drawing a distinction between the competent and powerful role of the professional and the helplessness and passivity implied by the term 'patient'. This is just one example of many **dichotomies** in which the world is construed as a series of polar opposites, including the notion of being mentally healthy or mentally unwell, where one precludes the other and the line between is clearly established.

Dichotomies
divisions into two parts, often seen as opposing.

Such a process has been seen to maintain systems of inequality and contribute to powerlessness rather than empowerment. Holley, commenting on her own experience as a service user, states that 'all professionals, (whatever their discipline, from psychiatrist to social worker), are not a different species to those they care for. In fact everyone is on the mental health continuum . . . so called mental "illness" is unequivocally part and parcel of the human condition, and less of an abnormality' (2008: 151). The challenge of working within an approach embedded within a shared humanity is one to which we will return later in this chapter and throughout the book.

Voices from the Past

Despite what might be seen as the relatively recent emergence of the service user 'voice' and movement, examples of people speaking out about their experiences of mental distress and the treatment they have received can be found throughout history. The difference is likely to be seen in the extent to which such expressions were seen as lone and individual voices, rather than as part of wider networks of interconnecting experiences within and across national boundaries and, increasingly, making effective use of the mass media and the internet to communicate and campaign. The extent to which the voices of people who have experienced mental distress have been recognized and heard, however, has to be assessed against the preponderance of both professional and 'lay' or public perspectives (Foster, 2007).

Early examples of protest against inhumane treatment and enforced incarceration in Britain include 'The Petition of the Poor Distracted People in the House of Bethlem', sent to the House of Lords in 1620, and the efforts of the Alleged Lunatics' Friends Society set up by John Percival in 1845, drawing on his own experience of incarceration. The early twentieth century saw the founding of the National Society for Lunacy Law Reform and similar developments in North America, where Elizabeth Packard organized the Anti-Insane Asylum Society in 1896 after being committed by her husband. She was followed by Clifford Beers, who wrote an autobiographical account of his experiences in 1908 in *A Mind that Found Itself* and set up the National Committee on Mental Hygiene, later to become the National Mental Health Association (Fennell, 1996; Crossley, 2006). Such examples led Campbell

(1996) to point out that there has always been evidence of protest and challenge regarding the quality of care and treatment offered.

Such activities have also been accompanied by a range of literature and autobiographical writing detailing the experiences of distress that continues today, from the nineteenth-century work of Charlotte Perkins Gilman (2009) and the poetry of John Clare to that of Wilfred Owen in the aftermath of the First World War, and the writing of Sylvia Plath and Susanna Kaysen (1995), to name but a few examples. Plath's account of her experiences in her 1963 novel *The Bell Jar* uses the metaphor in the title of the book to explain her own breakdown, and Kaysen describes the ease with which one can slip into a 'parallel universe' where, she says:

> the laws of physics are suspended. What goes up does not necessarily come down; a body at rest does not tend to stay at rest; and not every action can be counted on to provoke an equal and opposite reaction. Time, too, is different. It may run in circles, flow backward, skip about from now to then. The very arrangement of molecules is fluid: Tables can be clocks; faces, flowers.   (1995: 6)

Janet Frame's work (for example, Frame 2000) has drawn considerably on her own experiences, as has that of Clare Allen, who has written a regular column in the *Guardian* and also satirized her own experiences in her 2009 novel *Poppy Shakespeare*. Films from *One Flew Over a Cuckoo's Nest* to *Girl Interrupted* and *A Beautiful Mind* may also provide a partial insight into people's experiences of mental distress and their use of services.

Activity

Read a book or watch a film that refers to the experience of mental ill health. Think about the content in relation to the messages it may offer in terms of the perspective on the mental health experience of the individual(s) concerned. If possible, share your views and ideas with others who have read or watched the same or alternative books or films.

Ask yourself the following questions:

• To what extent does this book or film reflect the historical context in which it was produced?
• Does the book or film offer any positive messages?
• Is the material presented from any particular perspective(s), and if so, are there any obvious gaps in the views as they are presented?

The use of literature, film and other media such as the internet, for instance by blogging, is increasingly recognized as a valuable source of material in understanding human experience and in contributing to professional education across a range of health and social care professions. When reading or viewing such accounts, however, it is necessary to reflect on the range and diversity of experiences that are presented. There is a danger that messages of disempowerment may be reinscribed and that powerful messages that run counter to the prevailing discourse may be overlooked. This might include the recognition that, for some individuals, there may be comforting, creative or other positive experiences associated with hearing voices or the feeling of being 'high': 'It's like having company in your head . . . that you've always got someone with you' (quoted from an interview in Foster, 2007: 93).

The service user movement: consumers, citizens and activists

Although the term 'service user movement' is often used and offers a convenient general description of a range of activities, the concept itself is complex, containing many diverse objectives, opinions and activities, ranging from questioning the concept of mental illness to the organized involvement of users and carers in existing systems of mental health care, whether in relation to policy and service design or to delivery and evaluation. Similarly, whilst this section of the chapter will explore consumerism, citizenship and activism in turn, in practice the boundaries between these concepts may be disputed and blurred.

The birth of the service user 'movement' as it is currently understood is generally agreed to have occurred in the latter part of the twentieth century with a number of developments in Britain and more widely across Western Europe. These were fuelled by a complex mix of factors: Barnes and Bowl (2001: 30) refer to radical critiques of psychiatry and the welfare state by professionals, an increasing concern for civil rights, an emphasis on consumer rights and information, growing interest in self-help, media attention to abuses within large institutions and hospitals and the influence of social and political movements, including the women's movement and campaigns for gay liberation.

Internationally, a number of organizations exist with varying degrees of collaboration between survivors and professionals. Some groups were initially the preserve of those who had not experienced mental health difficulties themselves, and it is only over time that the voices of survivors have increasingly begun to take centre stage. A meeting of the World Federation of Mental Health in 1982 established, with the involvement of Judi Chamberlin as a consumer-advocate, that 'It could no longer be taken for granted that the rules of therapeutic interaction would be laid down by society's designated helpers without a dialog with the help-seekers' (Brody, 1998: 129). Efforts were also initiated in New Zealand by Mary O'Hagan to develop a global organization of survivors in the World Federation of Psychiatric Users (WFPU), which was formally established in 1991.

Consumerism

As self-help became legitimized within the psychiatric establishment, many user-initiated developments began to be seen as examples of reformist consumerism. Concerns were raised that there was a focus primarily on 'co-operative consumers', with Chamberlin stating that 'The very term "consumers" implies an equality of power which simply does not exist; mental health "consumers" are still subject to involuntary commitment and treatment, and the defining of their experience by others' (1990: 333–4). In referring to the growth and influence of consumerism, Campbell points out that there is 'a considerable difference between valuing a madperson as a consumer or recipient of mental health services and valuing a madperson as a contributing and insightful member of society' (1996: 220). His comments point to the distinction between varying levels of involvement and the ambition of the agenda of any particular group or campaign. The former is now clearly embedded within legislation in the UK and many other countries, with requirements from the 1990 Community Care Act onwards referring to the need to involve service users and carers in planning services. The Health and Social Care Act 2001 provides for service user involvement at a strategic level as a legal requirement, and the Department of Health (2006) White Paper, *Our Health, Our Care, Our Say*, emphasizes the need for more choice and louder voice for users of health care services alongside better prevention, tackling inequality, improving access to services and more support for people with long-term needs.

There is, however, a distinction to be drawn between the opportunity to provide feedback on a service or a collaborative approach to assessment and planning, as useful as this may be, and the right to participate actively in shaping services. Not least is the question of who holds the power and the extent to which feedback or choice are not only listened to but acted upon by professionals and services. In this respect, Hugman cautions that 'The very existence of occupations which make claims to expertise in areas of health and welfare may be said to have been founded on the exclusion of users from the definition of need or appropriate responses to its remedy' (1998: 137).

The implications of applying a consumerist agenda, originally developed within the world of the marketplace, to health and welfare settings also has implications for those working in the sector. If service users are consumers then professionals are seen as producers and the service as a product. The right to an assessment does not guarantee a service, and professionals are increasingly caught up in a culture of targets, performance indicators and the gatekeeping of scarce resources at the expense of building relationships and a broader professional response to distress or disadvantage. In discussing the limitation of applying a consumerist model to mental health services, with their potential for coercion, one service user with experience of inpatient care scathingly compared users' 'consumption' of mental health services to 'the consumption of Rentokil by cockroaches' (Barker & Peck, 1987: 1).

Even within this more limited agenda there is still a long way to go. The *Fifth Annual Survey of Community Mental Health Service Users* (Healthcare Commission, 2008) found that only 59 per cent had received a copy of their care plan and that 45 per cent had not had a care review in the past year. Additionally, 24 per cent said that they had not been involved in deciding what went into their care plan and 16 per cent said that their diagnosis had not been discussed with them. Others have critiqued the consumerist model of user involvement as being potentially 'regressive' (Beresford, 2003) and as representing the 'commodification of welfare' (Cowden & Singh, 2007: 5) within an agenda which is only superficially progressive.

Citizenship

The term 'citizen' is described by Lester and Glasby as incorporating 'a cluster of meanings including defined legal and social status; a means of signifying political identity; a focus of loyalty; a requirement to perform duties; expectations of rights; and a yardstick of behaviour' (2006: 156). For many people, using mental health services has been instrumental in the removal or denial of many aspects of citizenship. This includes the actual experience of hospitalization and/or treatment as well as exclusion and discrimination more generally within society. As a consequence, increasing attention has been paid to an agenda emphasizing political rights and a shift in the balance of power between service users and professionals.

There are risks, however, that the wider discourse of social inclusion obscures the reality that a failure to conform will result in exclusion. Notions of responsibilities accompanying rights could be narrowly interpreted as needing to comply with treatment or to curb 'unusual' behaviours, thereby signalling conformity and compliance with conventionally accepted norms.

Notwithstanding such concerns, the current focus on citizenship does offer potential advantages in terms of involvement in decision-making, both for individuals in respect of their own care, and for greater opportunities to influence the design and delivery of services. More fundamentally, notions of citizenship have the potential to move us beyond the narrow confines of increasing user involvement in relation to services alone, as beneficial as this may be, to challenging wider systems of power and inequality within which discrimination and exclusion are currently maintained. Barnes and Bowl (2001) relate such an approach to the concept of empowerment, which can be understood as either reactive or proactive, respectively describing the relationship between service user and service provider or acting on broader systems of power. Proactive empowerment can also be seen to offer opportunities for building alliances with other disenfranchised groups, creating partnerships to challenge discrimination and exclusion (Sayce, 2000; Lester & Glasby, 2006).

Activism

Moving to the other end of the spectrum, professionals are sidelined within the more radical edge groups such as the European Network of (ex-)Users and Survivors of Psychiatry, which includes groups from the UK such as the Hearing Voices Network, MindLInk and VOX (Voices of Experience) in Scotland and the Irish Advocacy Network. The purpose of the network is to 'support each other in the personal, political and social struggle against expulsion, injustice and stigma in our respective countries' and 'promote and improve the human rights of (ex-)users and survivors of psychiatry; to fight for (ex-)user/survivor controlled alternatives to psychiatry and against abuse and coercion' (ENUSP, 2009). Such groups are more likely to challenge the very meaning of 'mental illness' as a social construction and to campaign actively for an end to discrimination and abuse in terms of human rights in society, rather than working to improve existing services. Mad Pride sees parallels with the Gay Pride movement, and its very name demonstrates the reclaiming of the language historically associated with shame and stigma. Similarly, other groups such as Survivors Speak Out and the UK Advocacy Network (UKAN) campaign for people to have their voices heard and to have an increasing say over their lives whilst acknowledging the benefits of working alongside other voluntary sector organizations (Crepaz-Keay, 2008).

Service User Involvement

To return to service user involvement, however, what is clear from reviewing the level of user involvement across a range of organizations and settings is the need to examine the extent to which this remains tokenistic or is more fundamental in its approach. Arnstein's ladder of participation (1969; see Figure 1.1) is still frequently referred to in identifying various levels of involvement and participation and to assist in developing a greater degree of community participation. One of the crucial factors to be taken into consideration is the extent to which service users are involved in setting the agenda rather than responding to an agenda that has already been determined by others.

Reflection point

Using the ladder of participation, think of any organization or group that you are aware of and consider the level of involvement and participation in it.
- If you consider that this is not at the maximum, identify some actions that might help to increase it.
- Think about the ways in which social workers may be able to increase levels of involvement.
- What might be some of the barriers to increasing involvement and how could these be overcome?

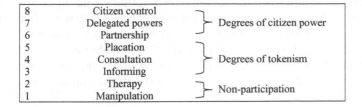

Figure 1.1   Arnstein's ladder of participation
Source: Arnstein (1969: 247)

Despite the inclusion of service user involvement in many policies and guidance documents, concerns continue that meaningful involvement remains limited. Paradoxically this may be hindered by the increasing levels of monitoring and regulation which require highly professionalized responses and leave service user involvement as a tick-box criterion. However, it is possible to find ways of increasing participation (see 'Practice example').

Practice example

A voluntary sector organization was set up in the early 1980s to provide alternatives to statutory mental health services within an area where access to services and support on a 24/7 basis was limited. In particular, local mental health workers, social workers and other community activists were aware of the shortfall in provision and worked together to initiate this development. The organization began with limited finances, and with a small number of staff and some volunteers began to provide weekend support, social activities and group home accommodation. Over a number of years the organization grew, with increased staff numbers and funding, becoming part of a highly professionalized sector commissioning services with the local social services and health agencies. Today the agency is involved in providing community-based services including housing support, drop-ins and community development projects, with a particular emphasis on the mental health and wellbeing of Black and minority ethnic communities. This level of organization requires a supportive infrastructure and high-quality leadership, with an executive director and a management committee.

The challenge now for an organization such as this is to increase the level of participation of its members in a number of ways, moving towards an organization that is user led. The development of a service user involvement group with its own newsletter and meetings is the first step in increasing participation, and this also provides support for those members who sit on the management committee. The development of quality standards and monitoring and review systems within the organization is also involving service users, who have received training and increasingly take a lead in this activity. Building on this experience, some of the service users have also recently been commissioned to undertake a service user evaluation of an educational programme providing training for Approved Mental Health Professionals at a local university.

What will be evident from this example is that there is no quick and easy way to make the shift to a user-led organization. However, it is possible to see that each small step in the process may help move the organization forward. It may also be worth acknowledging that were such a development to begin now – that is, twenty-five years later – the importance of user and carer involvement at the beginning would be non-negotiable.

Other examples of the ways in which service users are increasingly involved in services include developments in practice, education and research.

Practice

There are a number of examples of specially designated posts for service users in mental health teams, recognizing the valuable contribution of a service user perspective in enhancing the way in which care and support is offered.

It is also important to remember that there are already many people working in mental health services who have themselves experienced mental health difficulties. The opportunities for sharing this experience with colleagues will depend on the safety and level of open discussion within any one team, but such sharing has the potential to contribute to challenging 'them and us' attitudes (see 'Practice example').

Practice example

Malcolm had been involved with mental health services for many years and his confidence and hope for the future were at a low level. Having received a letter from a service user involvement team in the local NHS Trust, he asked his social worker for more information about who had sent the letter. He was surprised and clearly pleased to learn that service users like himself were employed within the organization, and this prompted further discussion about his own plans for recovery.

Education

Within education, particularly professional training courses for social work and health care professionals, there has been a slow but increasing level of involvement of service users/survivors, ranging from the one-off lecture through offering a service user perspective to the embedding of a more systematic approach to user involvement throughout the design, development, delivery and evaluation of modules and courses. Despite this, Livingston and Cooper (2004) estimated that there were only two user/academic teaching and research posts in the UK.

Research

The involvement of service users and carers in research has become embedded within policy guidance (Department of Health, 1999c, 2001c), although progress is variable, ranging from none through consultation and involvement to user-led or user-controlled research. Examples of user-led or user-controlled research include the Strategies for Living project undertaken by the Mental Health Foundation, the work of the Service User Research Enterprise (SURE) unit associated with the Institute of Psychiatry, and the Sainsbury Centre for Mental Health's User-Focused Monitoring (Rose et al., 1998).

Beresford (2000), drawing on his experience as a service user, an activist in the service user movement and a professor of social policy, highlights the way that service user knowledges can offer a challenge to the dominant discourse within mainstream mental health theory and research, being based on direct and personal experiences. Similarly, Rose, in discussing user involvement in research, argues that 'entry of the bearers of unreason into rational polity is another way in which madness strikes back' (2008: 639). Rose goes on to point out that the description of 'user researcher' is not an additive concept but a 'double identity' (p. 640), in which the experience of mental health services contributes directly to practice. The tensions that may arise in this process are addressed by Rose and others (Trivedi & Wykes, 2002; Telford & Faulkner, 2004). However, there remains a sense that, despite the challenges involved and the very real costs in time and money, there are tangible benefits to be found in the development of new research areas, and a greater emphasis on accessible research design and dissemination.

Future challenges

User involvement in mental health continues to offer a significant challenge, as can be seen from the foregoing discussion. Not least important is the need to overcome the deficit model, attributed to illness, in which the very nature of mental distress is used as a justification for exclusion or for silencing the voices of experience. The alternative recognizes the need to address the structural inequalities which McDaid sees as the real barrier to participation. She proposes that an Equality of Conditions Framework provides 'a lens through which one can identify the full range of social disadvantages faced by mental health service users' (2009: 464), and points to the need to tackle the inequalities in power and resources which undermine meaningful involvement, including a lack of respect and recognition for service users' experiences and knowledge, isolation and unequal access to technical or procedural knowledge. This perspective can also be seen to overturn consumer welfarist notions of involvement in which participation is seen to increase power, and offers, in its place, a more fundamental rethinking of power as a prerequisite for involvement.

Evidence to demonstrate the successful impact of involvement is, as yet, limited and is often preoccupied with the therapeutic impact on the service users themselves, rather than their influence on existing systems, decisions and priorities. Whilst such intrinsic factors are in themselves valuable and may in turn influence the effectiveness of involvement and participation, such as enhanced confidence leading to increasing involvement, there is a need for further work to be undertaken to increase our understanding of the outcomes as well as the process of service user participation (Carr, 2004; Doel et al., 2007).

Recovery

The concept of recovery has come to be of central importance in much of the user/survivor literature and also in underpinning and informing contemporary services. However, despite its widespread appeal and acclaim it is necessary to interrogate and explore the term and its application critically.

Conventionally, 'recovery' has been a term associated with freedom from symptoms and a return to health and wellbeing, frequently described as being 'back to normal'. In the past, a diagnosis of schizophrenia was associated with the advice to individuals that they would need care and treatment for the rest of their lives and would be unlikely to work: in other words, recovery was not thought possible. Such advice was framed or constructed within a medical model of illness, offering little hope of improvement. Coleman describes his experience:

> It was if the system had no expectation of me recovering, instead the emphasis was on maintenance. I am not saying that those who worked in the system did not care for me, they did. They clothed me, fed me, housed me and ensured that I took my medication. What they did not do was consider the possibility that I could return to being the person I once was.   (1999: 5)

As already suggested, it is necessary to look critically at the way in which any ideas are considered within a dichotomous framework, in this case, the temptation to fall into a 'bad' psychiatry versus 'good' 'user' debate. Instead we need to recognize the various and diverse meanings of recovery within the service user world, and also to recognize the potential for more nuanced responses from professionals and others working within mental health services.

There are many different definitions and stories of recovery that can be found within the literature. These include the work of Pat Deegan (1996), who refers to the concept of recovery as follows:

> Recovery does not refer to an end product or result. It does not mean that one is 'cured' or simply stabilised or maintained in the community. Recovery often involves a transformation of the self wherein one

both accepts one's limitation and discovers a new world of possibility . . . This is the paradox of recovery i.e. that in accepting what we
cannot do or be, we begin to discover who we can be and what we
can do. Thus recovery is a process. It is a way of life. It is an attitude
and a way of approaching the day's challenges.

O'Hagan's writing (1999) also highlights the unique and highly personal nature of recovery for herself and many others, in her statement
that: 'Ultimately, recovery is something of a mystery to me, my own
included. I really can't tell you about its source because it comes from
the unnameable core of the human spirit.'

Attitudes towards services also vary enormously between those
service users that choose to work collaboratively with mental health
professionals to promote an agenda of recovery and those that prefer
to emphasize the importance of self-help. In Britain many service
users have been involved in the 'Experts by Experience' programme
initiated by the Department of Health, working to embed recovery
principles within mental health policy, guidance and service delivery.
In England this has led to a *Guiding Statement on Recovery* which
brings together a broad vision of recovery that 'involves a process of
changing one's orientation and behaviour from a negative focus on
a troubling event, condition or circumstance to the positive restora-
tion, rebuilding, reclaiming or taking control of one's life' (National
Institute for Mental Health in England, 2005a). Others, however, such
as Coleman (1999), understand recovery as a process of reclaiming
personal power and are critical of models of clinical and social recovery that continue to be located within the mental health system.

Notwithstanding the seemingly all-round wholesomeness of 'recovery', there remain continuing concerns as to the way in which the
concept is understood and applied. Deegan (2003) points to questions
regarding the extent to which it is being seen as relevant to everyone
experiencing mental health difficulties, whilst also pointing out the
dangers of recovery being oversimplified to a 'one size fits all' phenom-
enon. Deegan also raises a concern that the association of the recovery
movement with 'celebrity' may lead to questions about whether recovery is more of a myth than a reality. Additionally, there may also be
risks of political expediency in embracing a philosophy that has the
potential to be used to justify cuts in community-based services such
as day centres. This may be associated with a sanitized or 'watered
down' version of recovery which fails to challenge issues of inequality
and power. The close association of recovery with the importance of
personal stories or 'narratives' also positions recovery within a postmodern context and indicates that we should be aware of the risks as
well as the benefits inherent within it.

Despite these concerns, the recovery paradigm remains a central
principle for social work practice in mental health. In respect of this it
may be helpful to note O'Hagan's (1999) 'challenges' to promote the
notion of recovery within mental health services, which draw on her

experiences in New Zealand, offering parallels with work to promote partnership, participation and protection for Maori and Pacific peoples:

1. Assist us in reaching our own understanding of our illness or distress;
2. Encourage us to have hope;
3. Give us respect, rights and equality;
4. Only provide treatments and support that will reduce distress;
5. Enable us to use our own resourcefulness;
6. Facilitate our inclusion in our communities and cultures.

As O'Hagan also notes, these challenges require the involvement of three players: people with mental health difficulties themselves; their families and communities; and mental health services. We shall return to these three elements when considering practice in a later chapter. In the meantime it may be helpful simply to emphasize the importance of developing social work practice that promotes social inclusion and facilitates access to communities, and to use models of assessment, planning and intervention that support such an approach.

Carers

In moving on to consider carers' experiences, some brief discussion concerning the relationship between users and carers is required. Whilst in some areas there may be overlaps in terms of shared issues, in others the experiences of carers will be entirely separate and unique to the role of being a carer, with the possibility that in some circumstances, the interests and views of users and carers will be in opposition.

There may also be some ambivalence regarding being seen as a carer in terms of the implications this has for other dimensions of existing relationships and notions of reciprocity. Bucknall and Holmes point out that 'if there is a group of people called carers, then there must also be a corresponding group who need care (the cared for)' (2001: 127). Being viewed as a carer may also sit uncomfortably alongside other relationships, such as being a partner. In rejecting the label of 'carer', Sayce (2000) comments on the importance of mutual relationships rather than care being simply a one-way transaction. In this sense the 'carer/cared for' distinction also negates the positive contribution that can be made by the individual seen as having a mental health problem. Whilst acknowledging these conceptual difficulties, the term 'carer' will be used in this text as a convenient way of describing those who provide care and support to someone close to them.

Although a number of accounts of carers' experiences have challenged the negative use of the term 'burden' in respect of their caring responsibilities, there are undoubtedly a number of issues and concerns associated with the role of being a carer. Some of the difficulties faced by many family members and friends who provide care for someone, whether as a result of poor mental health, physical impairment or other health condition, include accessing information and support, feeling marginal or being viewed as interfering. An additional and significant factor in considering the challenges faced by carers in relation to mental health lies in the historical attitudes towards the relationship between the family and mental illness. Such attitudes have their origins in the view that damaging early family relationships are the cause of mental ill health, supported by the work of Laing (1965) and sociological critiques of the family. This was fuelled further by research into high levels of expressed emotion within families and findings linking these with higher rates of relapse in schizophrenia (Leff & Vaughan, 1981; Dixon & Lehman, 1995). Attempts to reconcile these views with the potential benefits of working with families have resulted in some complex linguistic manoeuvres in which the part played by family members in relapse is emphasized, whilst discussion of causation is avoided (Johnstone, 2000). Although it is vital that the negative family and relationship experiences of some mental health service users are heard and acknowledged, it is also necessary to avoid making judgements about all families and responding as if family members are the cause of the problems rather than having the potential to be part of the solution.

Carers' views and experiences need to be valued and recognized by professionals who will involve them as equal and expert partners in the provision of care and support. At the same time, it is likely that many issues will require careful and sensitive negotiation in terms of identifying the extent to which these interests align with those of the individual service user. In particular, aspects of confidentiality can highlight potential difficulties where the interests of the service user need to be paramount. Views regarding the capacity and resources of the service user may also not be in accord with others' opinions.

At the same time there are the very legitimate needs of carers themselves for support, recognizing the impact that caring may have on physical and emotional wellbeing. These needs have increasingly been recognized within policy and legislation, leading to the development of separate services and organizations offering carer support, not directly connected to mainstream mental health services. Further discussion regarding policy and practice will be addressed in later chapters, recognizing the importance of such issues and the need for careful consideration of the various interests involved.

Concluding Comments

This chapter has offered a brief introduction to some key issues regarding the experiences of service users and various aspects of service user involvement. The interests of carers have also been acknowledged, recognizing that at times these may diverge from those of service users.

Further Reading

Barnes, M. & Bowl, R. (2001) *Taking Over the Asylum*. Basingstoke: Palgrave

Sayce, L. (2000) *From Psychiatric Patient to Citizen*. Basingstoke: Macmillan

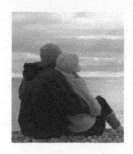

2 Theories, Models and Concepts

Key points

- Critical understanding of different models of mental health
- The influence of Western psychiatry and the 'medical model'
- The importance of religion and spirituality
- The contribution of a social perspective in promoting recovery

Introduction

What do we understand by the term 'mental health' and what characterizes the different theoretical models and concepts that are used to explain the causes and make sense of mental health difficulties? Why is it important for social workers to consider these issues?

This chapter will set out to answer these questions, exploring some of the key approaches to mental health and considering the implications of these for social work. Drawing on a critical social work perspective, the simplistic binary divide that is often presented between nature and nurture or medical and social models will be challenged. In their place a holistic and multifactorial model will be offered as a basis to inform and develop practice.

Theories and Models in Mental Health

We will begin by introducing some of the terms that will be found in this chapter. At its most straightforward, a theory seeks to explain and helps us to make sense of something, and a model is an attempt to describe something, sometimes becoming a building block of a larger theoretical framework. As Thompson (1995: 21) points out, a model tells us the 'how', whereas a theory tells us 'why'.

An example of a model can be found in the work of Goldberg and Huxley (1992), which describes the prevalence of mental disorders within the general population and considers the process involved in terms of an individual's journey from GP consultations through to outpatient and inpatient services. The model identifies a series of filters that operate between each stage of this journey, recognizing the influence of factors such as age, gender and class. However, this is clearly a model rather than a theory as, whilst there is a description or

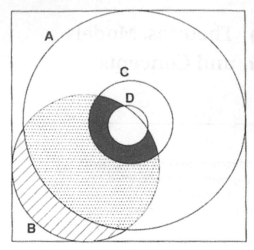

A = Consult their doctor during year

B = Episode of psychological distress during year (level 1)

C = Identified by their doctor as psychiatrically ill (level 3)

D = Referred to mental illness services (level 4)

▨ Do not pass 1st filter (ill, but do not consult)

⠿ Do not pass 2nd filter (illness not recognised by Dr)

■ Do not pass 3rd filter (not referred to mental illness services)

Figure 2.1 Venn diagram showing the relationship of disorders at different levels. The square represents the population at risk
Source: Goldberg and Huxley (1992: 6, fig. 1.1)

mapping of the processes involved, this does not necessarily tell us why these things happen.

Goldberg and Huxley's diagram of the model is shown in Figure 2.1, as this also helps to illustrate the importance of a broader understanding of mental health issues in social work and the prevalence of mental health problems within the wider community that social workers may encounter.

Whereas in the physical or natural sciences theory is seen both to explain and potentially to predict, the reality of theory within the social sciences, dealing with human actors and their behaviour, is rather more complex. Firstly, theories are used at a number of different levels and can be found to explain anything from the entire state of the world, as Marxist or feminist theories aim to do, to smaller-scale or everyday events, as micro-level theory does, with middle-range theory in between. Secondly, there is the question of the evidence used to support a theory: in strictly scientific terms a theory is testable and, if proven, allows predictions to be made. However, in the social world this is not feasible as it would be almost impossible to prove, for example, that social and environmental processes, such as the experience of poverty or abuse, were directly responsible for the development of mental health difficulties. Finally, there is the vital question of the political, economic and social context within which any theory is located.

The importance of professional practice underpinned by critical reflection points us towards a questioning stance on all theory, requiring us to revisit ideas, to examine multiple viewpoints and, where necessary, to challenge the theory that is presented. Aspects of this may include exploring the reasoning behind a theory, its political context or the methodology used to generate research evidence. An illustration of this can be found in the attention being paid to the importance of cognitive behavioural therapy in treating common mental health difficulties. Whilst there is a growing evidence base to support its use, there may also be elements of expediency in terms of its cost, since it is delivered by a range of staff trained for this one intervention, rather than by professionally trained – and costly – psychologists or psychotherapists. In turn of course, this expediency may also be a driver behind research priorities and funding.

Mental illness, mental health and wellbeing

A fundamental question concerns the relationship between mental illness and mental health, where frequently one is understood to be the absence of the other. If we take the view that mental illness is a disease or sickness requiring diagnosis and treatment within a medical framework, the explanation will often turn towards the issues of pathology or psychopathology, symptoms and symptom control. The following definition of mental illness would seem to apply here: 'Clinically recognisable patterns of psychological symptoms or behaviour causing acute or chronic ill health, personal distress or distress to others' (WHO, 1992). We can call this a **paradigm** or a particular way of interpreting the world. However, to see the presence of illness or health purely in terms of a simple dualism conceals rather than reveals the many different responses to the question of what mental health is.

Paradigm a conceptual framework that guides thinking and research within a particular set of beliefs.

In order to explore this further it is worth considering some of the responses that have been offered, beginning with a health promotion perspective, based on a continuum that takes into account resilience and coping factors as well as risks and pathology. The following definition of mental health illustrates this: 'Mental health is the emotional and spiritual resilience which enable us to enjoy life and survive pain, disappointment and sadness. It is a positive sense of well-being and an underlying belief in our own and other's dignity and worth' (Health Education Authority, 1997).

The term 'mental wellbeing' has also come into use, linked to 'mental capital', as a resource that needs nurturing if society is to prosper. The definition of mental capital used by the Foresight Report is as follows:

> encompassing a person's cognitive and emotional resources. It includes their cognitive ability, how flexible and efficient they are at learning and their 'emotional intelligence', such as their social skills and resilience in the face of stress. It therefore conditions how well an individual is able to contribute effectively to society, and also to experience a high personal quality of life.

The report also defines mental wellbeing, as:

> a dynamic state in which the individual is able to develop their potential, work productively and creatively, building strong and positive relationships with others and contribute to their community.

> It is enhanced when an individual is able to fulfil their personal and social goals and achieve a sense of purpose in society.
> (Foresight Mental Capacity and Wellbeing Project, 2008: 10)

The report, written by an independent group to inform government thinking and policy, emphasizes that mental capital and wellbeing are closely linked and that it is both 'challenging and natural' to think of the mind in a similar way to that in which one would think of financial capital.

Reflection point

Compare the definitions of mental health and wellbeing above.
Consider the implications of each and evaluate the perspective that underpins it.
How do these definitions relate to the purpose and values of social work?

Within the health promotion literature the term *salutogenesis* (Antonovsky, 1987) is used to acknowledge the rich and dynamic complexity of human life and movement towards health, building on opportunities to promote resilience and coping strategies rather than a narrow focus on pathology and treatment. Remaining within a health promotion approach, MacDonald and O'Hara's Ten Element Map (1998), set out in Figure 2.2, identifies how different factors may promote or undermine mental health, with those above the dotted line acting to promote and those below the line to demote mental health.

An important aspect of this model is that in addition to acknowledging the complex interaction and inter-relatedness of each element, each can be considered at micro, meso and macro levels, recognizing individual, institutional and societal influences. For example, when applying this model to the mental health of older people we might

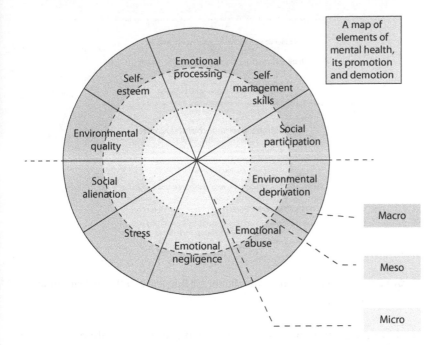

Figure 2.2 MacDonald and O'Hara's Ten Element Map
Source: MacDonald and O'Hara (1998), reproduced in Cattan and Tilford (2006: 22)

need to acknowledge negative societal attitudes to ageing and the impact of these on self-esteem, along with increasing social isolation, failing physical health and, for many, the impact of poverty and loneliness.

Such a model would appear to complement a social work perspective, drawing on an ecological framework, such as the one in Figure 2.3, which recognizes and understands the 'complexity of any given situation and individual circumstance' (Baldwin & Walker, 2005: 40).

Another dimension also concerns the socio-cultural context within which any discussion about mental health is taking place. Attention is frequently focused on the fear and stigma which can underpin responses to mental illness, as, although many people are generally sympathetic, responses to the Department of Health Annual Surveys into Attitudes towards Mental Illness (TNS UK, 2010) found that a significant proportion would not want to live next door to someone with a mental illness, or thought that one of the main causes of mental illness was a lack of self-discipline and willpower. Critics of the essentialist nature of the medical model, incorporating notions of illness over which the person has no responsibility, see this as offering a 'toxic ensemble' (Read & Haslam, 2004: 141) which maintains the 'othering'

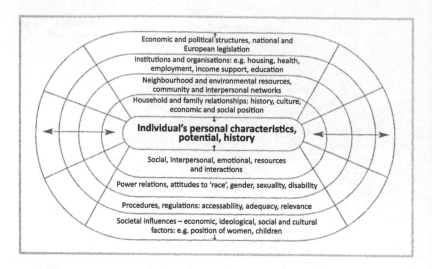

Economic and political structures, national and European legislation

Institutions and organisations: e.g. housing, health, employment, income support, education

Neighbourhood and environmental resources, community and interpersonal networks

Household and family relationships: history, culture, economic and social position

Individual's personal characteristics, potential, history

Social, interpersonal, emotional, resources and interactions

Power relations, attitudes to 'race', gender, sexuality, disability

Procedures, regulations: accessability, adequacy, relevance

Societal influences – economic, ideological, social and cultural factors: e.g. position of women, children

Figure 2.3   The web of interacting factors influencing individual situations
Source: Baldwin (2000)

of people experiencing mental health difficulties, fuelling prejudice and discrimination.

Negative attitudes may also influence the views of mental health professionals (Raskin & Lewandowski, 2000), as well as having a significant impact on those who themselves experience mental health difficulties, both practically and psychologically. Cooke (2008) describes the psychological consequences as including hopelessness, taking on the social role of a 'mental patient' and decreased ownership and agency, as well as having the potential to deny both positive and negative aspects of individuals' lived experience. Working to counter the damaging effects of stereotypical views relies on listening to service users' and survivors' experiences and the development of narratives of hope and recovery.

Looking back over time there are many different ways in which people have understood mental ill health. Evidence from early societies such as ancient Egypt suggests that people who might now be considered to be mentally ill received a range of treatments including sleep therapy and excursions on the Nile, and 'curative treatment' was attributed to the wearing of amulets or charms. In pre-industrial Britain, sickness in general was frequently understood in terms of divine retribution or the work of the devil, with such notions being rooted in the Old Testament (Read, 2004). Such ideas often led to the persecution of the sufferers themselves, and in some cases, that of those who tried to help them. The persecution of women healers and herbalists accused of witchcraft in attempting to heal the sick was also legitimized by witch-hunt manuals such as the 1486 *Malleus Malefi-carum* or 'Hammer of Evil-doers'.

It is also relevant here to acknowledge a wider global and international perspective on different approaches to mental health, recognizing that different world views, faiths and traditions continue to be a central element in people's understanding and responses.

The implications of these different approaches can be wide ranging. For example, are people experiencing mental health difficulties seen as blameworthy and responsible for their condition, unwell and in need of medical intervention, or in need of sanctuary and seclusion? More specifically, for social work, different understandings may influence whether or not the social worker has a role in promoting mental health, providing a rehabilitative approach in the wake of medical treatment, or as a key member of a multiprofessional team working to offer a range of psychological and social interventions as part of a broader package of care. This role may also encompass, at different times, the need to challenge stigma and discrimination, to work with families and carers as part of a wider system or undertaking an assessment for compulsory admission to hospital.

Notwithstanding the intention of this text to promote a social perspective on mental health and the valuable contribution that social work has to offer in this area, it is important that this chapter offers an introduction to a range of approaches, including the medical model, as well as considering a critique of this from a range of alternatives, before a holistic approach underpinned by a social perspective is proposed.

The Medical Model

In reality, the medical model is itself complex and at times contradictory, incorporating a number of different strands rather than offering one simple explanation. However, it is possible to view this as embedded within the development of science and medicine, which in Europe was especially associated with industrialization and the move from a rural to an urban economy. The shift from a pre-modern to a modern society was also accompanied by a decline in the influence of religion and the availability of increasingly rational and logical explanations for previously unexplainable phenomena. Increasing knowledge about mental illness and the development of psychiatry can be seen as reflecting other advances in scientific knowledge and medicine.

All of this provides a backdrop to an understanding of mental health based on the increasing power of the medical profession, supported by a scientific paradigm and continuing developments in treatment and cure. Broader issues of power and inequality can also be identified within this discourse, recognizing the privileging of male, White, European, able-bodied and heterosexual experience. This can be seen to have far-ranging implications, which will be considered in Chapter 6. Related to this, Fernando (2002) describes the 'culture of psychiatry', which reflects the particular historical and social context within which psychiatry developed, thereby determining who was acceptable and who was not, inherently incorporating racism (and sexism) and an assumed superiority of Western ways of thinking.

Overall, the term 'medical model' can be seen to incorporate the following features:

- a disease process;
- the influence of genetic, biological and or chemical factors;
- a response to illness based on diagnosis and treatment by professionals.

An early and highly influential example of the way in which thinking about mental illness developed can be found in Kraepelin's work in Germany in the late nineteenth century. Drawing on patient case studies, Kraepelin (1913) developed a system of psychiatric classification, based on the idea that there were an identifiable number of psychiatric disorders, each with its own **aetiology**, **pathology** and symptoms. He proposed that the identification and classification of symptoms would in time uncover the underlying cause of each condition. He was particularly interested in the early onset of symptoms of persecutory delusions and catatonia where there appeared to be a poor outcome, and drew these together into a diagnosis of 'dementia praecox', often referred to as 'senility of the young'. His lasting influence was to create a system of classification that underpins those in use today, based on the identification of illness through symptoms or 'function' rather than pathology.

Aetiology a term used to describe the origins of a particular condition or disease.

Pathology evidence of changes in the body indicating disease.

The two main classification systems in current use are the Diagnostic and Statistical Manual (DSM) (American Psychiatric Association, 1994), developed in the USA and currently in its fourth version, with a fifth planned for 2013, and the International Classification of Diseases (ICD), now in its tenth iteration (WHO, 1992). Whilst these systems continue to evolve, both are based on a medically oriented approach, as the following extract from the ICD demonstrates:

Schizophrenia

The normal requirement for a diagnosis of schizophrenia is that a minimum of one very clear symptom (and usually two or more if less clear-cut) belonging to any one of the groups listed as (a) to (d), or symptoms from at least two of the groups referred to as (e) to (h), should have been clearly present for most of the time during a period of 1 month or more.

Conditions meeting such symptomatic requirements but of duration less than 1 month (whether treated or not) should be diagnosed in the first instance as acute schizophrenia-like psychotic disorder (F23.2) and reclassified as schizophrenia if the symptoms persist for longer periods. Symptom (i) in the above list applies only to the diagnosis of Simple Schizophrenia (F20.6), and a duration of at least one year is required.

(a) thought echo, thought insertion or withdrawal, and thought broadcasting;

(b) delusions of control, influence, or passivity, clearly referred to body or limb movements or specific thoughts, actions, or sensations; delusional perception;

(c) hallucinatory voices giving a running commentary on the patient's behaviour, or discussing the patient among themselves, or other types of hallucinatory voices coming from some part of the body;

(d) persistent delusions of other kinds that are culturally inappropriate and completely impossible, such as religious or political identity, or superhuman powers and abilities (e.g. being able to control the weather, or being in communication with aliens from another world);

(e) persistent hallucinations in any modality, when accompanied either by fleeting or half-formed delusions without clear affective content, or by persistent over-valued ideas, or when occurring every day for weeks or months on end;

(f) breaks or interpolations in the train of thought, resulting in incoherence or irrelevant speech, or neologisms;

(g) catatonic behaviour, such as excitement, posturing, or waxy flexibility, negativism, mutism, and stupor;

(h) 'negative' symptoms such as marked apathy, paucity of speech, and blunting or incongruity of emotional responses, usually resulting in social withdrawal and lowering of social performance; it must be clear that these are not due to depression or to neuroleptic medication;

(i) a significant and consistent change in the overall quality of some aspects of personal behaviour, manifest as loss of interest, aimlessness, idleness, a self-absorbed attitude, and social withdrawal. (WHO, 1992)

This notion of classification, however, is not universally accepted and agreed, and questions continue to be asked about the reliability of diagnosis, meaning the extent to which there is agreement about symptoms and diagnosis between different groups of psychiatrists, both nationally and internationally. Responses to this range from continuing attempts to refine and improve these categories to challenges to the underlying notion of the 'holy grail'(Bentall, 2003: 65) by those who see the quest for classification itself as illusory (Read et al., 2004)

It is still relevant, however, for social workers at least to be aware of some of the key aspects of this framework. These can be summarized as follows.

Functional and organic disorders

A major distinction is drawn between functional and organic disorders, with the latter being recognized where underlying physical pathology is present. For example, this might include various forms of dementia where current scanning and imaging may be able to identify the particular changes that are taking place in the brain structure. Similarly, the damage associated with physical trauma or the long-term effects of alcohol use may be physically identifiable.

By comparison, functional illnesses are those where the illness is assumed from the behaviour or 'function' of the individual. This creates a circular loop in which the 'symptoms' are seen to indicate the diagnosis of disorder, which in turn defines the symptoms. For schizophrenia, symptoms are seen to include perceptual distortions such as visual or aural hallucinations and delusional thinking. Increasingly, however, the concept of 'schizophrenia' is being seen as in urgent need of reappraisal, with evidence suggesting the need for more complex interactional models to explain the experience of psychosis (Bentall, 2003; Read et al., 2004).

Neuroses and psychoses

A further distinction that is often made within functional disorders is that between neuroses and psychoses. Psychoses are seen to be caused by an underlying biological disturbance and include categories such as schizophrenia and manic depression, now more commonly referred to as bipolar disorder. Neuroses, often described as '*common mental health problems*', include conditions such as depression and anxiety that may cause distress and impact on day-to-day life but do not usually affect insight or involve perceptual problems such as hallucinations or hearing voices. Sometimes understood as problems of living, these will be explored further in Chapter 9, as the experiences of depression and anxiety are frequently encountered by social workers in any area of practice.

Personality disorders

The category of functional illness also includes personality disorders, described in the ICD-10 (WHO, 1992) as 'a severe disturbance in the character, logical condition and behavioural tendencies of the individual, usually involving several areas of the personality, and nearly always associated with considerable personal and social disruption'. In practice this diagnosis is highly problematic. There remains a strong moral or judgemental component in the diagnosis, frequently being attached to people who are seen to be difficult or demanding, and feeding into a 'cycle of rejection' and exclusion (Johnstone, 2008; Pilgrim, 2009). Working with people with personality disorders will be considered further in later chapters in relation to trauma (Chapter 9) and risk (Chapter 11).

The continuing influence of genetics?

Within the overall umbrella of the medical model there continues to be a strong emphasis on the influence of genetics in certain aspects of research into mental illness, especially schizophrenia and bipolar disorder. This can be found in research based on families, especially studies of identical twins, where the expectation would be that a higher incidence of illness would be found in both twins. Of course it is possible that the occurrence of illness within identical twins may equally be a result of similar upbringing or environment, so research has also focused on adoption studies where identical twins have been separated at birth and one has been raised away from their birth parents. However, in reviewing the evidence for a genetic basis for schizophrenia, Joseph (2004) concludes that this rests on an uncritical acceptance of the research, related to a reluctance to consider wider causes of mental ill health. At present there appears to be little evidence that there is any straightforward explanation in terms of a simple gene marker. The evidence available may one day offer a significant piece of the jigsaw, but is unlikely to offer the whole picture, and an interactionist, multifactorial approach is more likely to prevail.

It is interesting to note that an emphasis on genetics and 'poor breeding' was challenged for many by the events of the First World War, when large numbers of men, including officers, returning from the trauma of trench warfare, were clearly exhibiting many of the symptoms of mental illness, with shell shock and other conditions. The notion that it was a result of inferior genes was increasingly replaced by the idea that it was the experience of war that had brought about high levels of distress, leading to a growing interest in social psychiatry, a branch of psychiatry interested in the effect of interpersonal relationships and the wider environment on mental health.

Cause and treatment?

The treatments associated with an emphasis on a medical model can also be seen to reflect changing knowledge and understanding. The increasing involvement of medical superintendents in the nineteenth-century asylums promoted, at least in theory, a medical rather than a custodial regime, and led to the introduction of many treatments that now sound crude and primitive. As well as the routine practice of blood letting, cupping (using suction to bring blood to the surface of the skin) and the use of leeches, these included the revolving chair into which the patient was strapped and then spun at 100 revolutions a minute (Ashworth, 1975).

One breakthrough in medical science concerned the discovery in the late eighteenth century that *general paresis*, a deteriorating dementia-like condition, resulted from the effects of syphilis. This provided a continuing impetus for seeking out an underlying physical disease process in other forms of mental illness. The introduction of other therapies such as **insulin therapy**, **electroconvulsive therapy (ECT)** and **psychosurgery** during the first half of the twentieth century also maintained the momentum of the medical model, as did the introduction

Insulin therapy a treatment introduced in the 1930s but no longer in use, involving an insulin-induced coma. This was believed to reduce the symptoms of schizophrenia.

Electroconvulsive therapy (ECT) may still be used to treat severe forms of depression when no other interventions appear to be successful, but remains controversial. The treatment is administered with an anaesthetic and involves passing an electric shock through the brain to induce a seizure. The side effects may include long-term memory loss and confusion. ECT is subject to safeguards contained within the Mental Health Act 1983.

Psychosurgery may be referred to as neurosurgery and includes lobotomy or leucotomy. It is no longer widely used and is subject to legislative safeguards.

of new drugs, especially the major tranquillizers. The proliferation of pharmaceutical treatments for depression, frequently aimed at women, contributed to the medicalization of mental distress.

The medical model with its associated language and orientation continues to frame much of what is offered within conventional mental health services, although, as we shall discuss later, new ideas and thinking offer a significant challenge to both theory and practice, supported by current policy developments.

Variations on a (Medical) Theme

So far this discussion has focused on the notion of an underlying disease process and the associated diagnosis and treatments that may be offered. However, it is also possible to recognize the wider impact of a medical model as the profession of psychiatry has extended its remit to other areas beyond the purely physical. Additionally, the underlying discourse of the medical model can also be found in certain areas of psychology and other psychological approaches in the response to illness based on diagnosis and treatment by professionals.

Freud and psychoanalysis

For many people mental health relates to psychological functioning and matters of the mind rather than the body. This is often associated with Sigmund Freud and his work on the unconscious in affecting the emotions. Whilst this is clearly a very different way of understanding mental health, parallels can be drawn in the way that psychoanalysis was conducted and the conventional approach to the treating and diagnosis of illness, with an emphasis on the underlying pathology, diagnosis and treatment determined by the professional. Within this model, rather than the diagnostic terms of the medical model such as, for example, schizophrenia, alternative labelling might refer to 'psychopathology', 'schizoid personality' or 'defence mechanisms'.

There can be some confusion regarding the involvement of various professional disciplines in psychoanalysis or other psychological therapies. There is no necessity for a psychiatrist, a medical doctor who has specialized in psychiatry, to be trained in psychoanalysis, psychotherapy or any other psychological therapy, although some choose to undertake further professional development in this area. Clinical psychologists working in this area may or may not undertake specific training in psychological therapies, whilst psychotherapy training may include those from other professional backgrounds, including social work, as well as people without previous professional qualifications.

As with a biological understanding of mental ill health, it is important to acknowledge the context within which psychoanalysis developed and the extent to which it reflected prevailing norms and values, founded upon a model of 'normal' development and anchored in traditional gender and cultural expectations. Whilst this has been critiqued in terms of the impact of power and inequality, a legacy of oppressive thinking in both theory and practice lingers on in some areas. The effect of this will be examined further in Chapter 6.

It is also of interest to note that the development of psychiatric social work in the early twentieth century was heavily influenced by this approach, with an expectation that social workers working with adults as well as children and families, often located within child guidance clinics, would be well versed in identifying and addressing faulty or 'abnormal' functioning in children or their families.

The influence of psychology

Focusing on individual behaviour and experience, the discipline of psychology has frequently been associated with ideas about normality and, hence, abnormality. As such it has been associated with statistical notions of what is normal; in other words, the behaviours that are most commonly found in any given population – running the risk that those who do not demonstrate these behaviours will be seen as deviant or abnormal. However, it would be inaccurate to assume one homogeneous psychological perspective, and instead psychology has given rise to a range of ways of understanding mental ill health, including behaviourist and cognitive approaches, with varying degrees of alignment to a medical model.

The 'Growth Movement'

Unlike models of mental health which have highlighted underlying pathology, be it physical or psychological, other therapeutic modalities have emerged from a developmental perspective which emphasizes growth. These are not founded on notions of illness but instead emphasize potential and opportunity, often within a person-centred framework. A key figure in this area is Carl Rogers (2003), who is credited with the development of person-centred therapy. Other variations on this approach include gestalt and group therapies. Within these therapies there is a central emphasis on the core principles of congruence, empathy and unconditional positive regard, with these being seen as central to supporting people in finding their own solutions to difficulties.

A Sociological Perspective

The development of sociology and the wider social sciences has offered new insights into and perspectives on understanding mental health, many of which highlight issues of power and oppression. Much has been written in this area, so the discussion here will address social causation and social construction, before moving to consider the relevance of postmodernism.

Social causation

A classic example of social causation can be found in the original work of Brown and Harris (1978), who, in considering depression amongst women, recognized the significance of social factors in contributing to the cause of depression, factors such as caring for children under the age of five, the loss of a mother, lack of employment outside the home and the lack of a confiding relationship. It is significant, however, that the diagnostic concept of depression remained unquestioned.

Critiques of mental health which draw attention to the other social aspects of life have also developed in relation to the impact of racism, sexism and other aspects of oppression. Further attention will be paid to these issues in Part 2 of this text, as they form an important element in a social perspective; however, the key message is that factors such as inequality, the experience of violence, abuse or trauma such as domestic violence and sexual abuse, as well as the impact of economic factors, poor housing and poverty etc. may all contribute to poor mental health. Current policy initiatives and developments have increasingly legitimized this perspective, recognizing that the dynamics of inequality which may contribute to the development of mental health difficulties are also likely to impact on access to services and support as well as the quality of help that may be on offer (Department of Health, 2002b; National Institute for Mental Health in England, 2003; Wanless, 2004).

Whilst social work has in the past been associated with this wider sociological critique of mental health, there remains a tension in practice between an emphasis on individual and family approaches and the potential for work with communities, not helped by the loss of community development approaches in social work that were influential in the 1970s and 1980s. Wider issues about the current state of social work are relevant here, as on the one hand some social workers can feel increasingly marginalized vis-à-vis other professional groups – both within mental health services and more generally. At the same time, the influence of social work thinking and social perspectives can be found in current mental health policies and guidance such as *The Ten Essential Shared Capabilities* (National Institute for Mental Health in England/Sainsbury Centre for Mental Health Joint Workforce Support Unit, 2004).

Labelling theory

The power of diagnosis as a labelling process also demonstrates the way in which behaviours may be interpreted as mental ill health depending on the context in which they are understood. Labelling theory (Scheff, 1975; Hannigan, 1999) describes how the effect of giving someone a label may also be self-fulfilling in that their behaviour will respond accordingly. Whilst potentially useful in explaining how behaviours may be maintained, in that the individual learns how to play the part of a patient or someone with a mental illness, labelling theory offers little help in understanding the origins of the behaviour in question.

Reflection point

Consider how being given a diagnosis of schizophrenia may impact on how people see themselves and how their behaviour is viewed by others.

One study (Rosenhan, 1973) is frequently cited as demonstrating labelling theory. This involved students presenting themselves at a psychiatric hospital, reporting various symptoms and subsequently being admitted. These initial behaviours created a frame by which all other behaviour was understood, including requests for paper and pens to record what was happening to them being understood as the symptom of 'writing behaviour'. A more recent attempt to replicate this study has been challenged (Slater, 2004; Spitzer et al., 2005) and this work, whilst of interest, remains controversial.

Social constructivism (social constructionism)

Sometimes termed social constructionism, social constructivism challenges the idea that the nature of mental illness is uncontested. Instead, apparently fixed and dominant notions of mental disorder are examined for their role in reinscribing systems of power and oppression and hence viewed as subject to meanings that are fluid and dynamic. This can be seen to include the way in which certain behaviours which offer a challenge to the status quo, or represent attempts to survive or escape oppression, are themselves interpreted as indicators of illness. Examples include the nineteenth-century diagnosis of drapetomania, which was seen to be an illness that caused slaves to run away from their owners (Fernando, 2002); the use and abuse of psychiatry in the Soviet Union in the twentieth century to contain and control dissidents (Johnstone, 2000); and the diagnosis of homosexuality as a disease, which was only formally rectified with its removal from psychiatric classification systems in the latter part of the twentieth century (King & Bartlett, 1999).

Social realism

As Rogers and Pilgrim (2000) point out, the assumptions of social cau-sation and social constructionism are incompatible: the evidence base for social causation starts with the given that mental illness exists, whilst social constructivism challenges the very existence of mental illness. In attempting to reconcile these conflicting paradigms, Rogers and Pilgrim propose that an approach grounded in social realism enables the acknowledgement of the reality of mental health and the social factors that may contribute to mental ill health, whilst at the same time maintaining a critical perspective on the ways in which the meaning of mental illness is produced.

Postmodernism, the psy complex and Foucault

This critique of mental health as a socially constructed means of control can be seen to have been developed further by postmodernist thinkers who have challenged the grand narrative of modernistic thinking with its notions of continuing progress. With its roots in the horrors of the Holocaust and the challenge of starvation and poverty in the world, postmodern thinking can be seen to offer an alternative view to the notion that the relentless progress of science will offer solu-tions to major world problems.

For social workers there is a particular resonance to the ideas of postmodernism regarding the tension between care and control. What has been described as the **'psy complex'** (Ingleby, 1985; Rose, 1985) suggests that there is a need for increasing governance and control in society and that this is manifest in various mechanisms and processes, including that of social work itself, but also more widely in education, family life and health care (Parton & O'Byrne, 2000).

'psy complex' ideas and thinking about human behaviour contained within psychiatry, psychol-ogy and sociology.

An illustration of this within a mental health context can be found in the development of assertive outreach services, which from one perspective can be seen as a positive attempt to support people whose lives are chaotic and unable to fit into the usual structures of support and services. Alternatively, however, such services could be under-stood as an intrusive process for ensuring that people conform to meet the needs of services and comply with their medication etc. in order not to relapse. Of course, in true postmodern style, the answer may be that both dynamics are in operation.

Michel Foucault's work (1965) is of relevance here in two key areas. First, in relation to the notion of surveillance in society, his concept of the panopticon highlights the processes of observation that may be central to hospital or other institutional or custodial care, such as prisons. The concept is understood in terms of an analysis of power, demonstrated in the building design, enabling attendants to see patients at all times and resulting in patients' 'self-surveillance' even when they were not actually being physically observed. (A modern-day version of this might be the speed cameras that prompt drivers to slow down even if the camera is not actually functioning.)

Second, Foucault's work identifies the fact that power is not necessarily a one-way process but can be multidirectional. This challenges the traditional critique of psychiatry which sees power invested solely in the privileged realm of psychiatry. Instead Foucault draws attention to issues of resistance and enables the identification of the experiences of those experiencing distress and their strategies for protest and survival.

Post-psychiatry

Drawing on the work of Foucault and others, psychiatrists Bracken and Thomas have developed a critique of psychiatry that offers a challenge to what they have described as the 'monologue of reason about madness' (2005: 2). They see this as encapsulating a **positivist**, scientific and above all modernist discourse within which the technical expertise of professionals is applied to manage and control mental illness in an individual frame that is isolated from a wider social and cultural context. In its place they argue that, in order to understand the experiences associated with mental distress, it is necessary to consider the individual within a wider context, taking into account culture and history and the many influences that affect our lives. They describe this as a hermeneutic or interpretative process, suggesting that 'attempting to understand phenomena such as hearing voices, sadness, withdrawal, euphoria, obsessionality, self-harm, suicidal ideation, fearfulness, and so on by reference to neurotransmitters and DNA alone is akin to someone attempting to understand a painting by an artist such as Picasso by analysing the chemical composition of the pigments on the canvas' (Bracken & Thomas, 2005: 15).

Positivist an understanding of knowledge based on positivism – the view that the world can be understood by observation using the scientific methods derived from the natural sciences.

Such an approach requires taking into consideration a number of perspectives, not just that of the professional, and emphasizes the rights of service users themselves to define their own reality. Bracken and Thomas have worked to apply this to their own practice by working closely with service user groups in promoting an agenda for citizenship, supporting the development of alternatives to conventional psychiatric care, including home treatment and community development based on the idea of 'safe spaces' within which people can explore their own understandings.

Other Ways of Understanding Mental Health Based on Individual Experience

Drawing on Foucault's thinking and that of other postmodern theorists, there is a need to avoid a tendency towards neat and orderly ways of understanding and making sense of mental health. The development of interest in individual narratives can also be linked to the increased interest in spirituality and mental health and, more generally, ideas of recovery. Linked to this, it is important to recognize the role that faith and religion have played in the many ways in which people have made sense of mental health and illness. This includes acknowledging both the positive aspects of acceptance and understanding that many find from organized religion and the stigma and exclusion experienced by others.

Recovery

As has already been discussed in the previous chapter, the term 'recovery' owes its origins to the service user movement (Deegan, 1988; Anthony, 1993), although is widely recognized and adopted within mainstream mental health services (Care Sector Improvement Partnership/Royal College of Psychiatrists/Social Care Institute for Excellence, 2007). Its adoption as a core underpinning concept in mental health practice and services could be viewed as demonstrating the extent to which service user perspectives are now placed centre stage, although, paradoxically, its widespread use could potentially undermine its power and meaning.

A definition from the service user literature describes recovery as 'a process, a way of life, an attitude, and a way of approaching the day's challenges. It is not a perfectly linear process ... Recovery has its seasons, its time of downward growth into darkness to secure new roots, and then times of breaking out into the sunlight' (Deegan, 1996). The issue of control is also emphasized by Double (2002): 'Recovery is about reclaiming a socially valued lifestyle and social empowerment. It means a person becoming in control of the decisions he or she takes.'

Key elements of recovery can therefore be seen to include the sense of a process rather than an end point, most effectively described by individuals in terms of their own experience or journey; it is not dependent on notions of 'cure' and is inextricably tied into notions of choice and self-determination. Furthermore, central to the idea of recovery is hope, something that for many people has been missing from their experience of mental illness, their encounters with others and their use of mental health services. The idea that life could get better, rather than worse, and the importance of a positive vision for the future has, in the past, been undermined by the negative associations of mental ill health embedded within individual attitudes and behaviour as well as institutional policies and practices. In attempting to reverse this negative cycle, Bassett and Repper also emphasize the point that 'hopeful workers are more likely to inspire hope in others' (2005: 16).

Spirituality

A belief in the uniqueness of each individual and an emphasis on a holistic perspective as an alternative to the mind–body dichotomy lies at the heart of thinking about spirituality and mental health, as the following definition from the National Spirituality and Mental Health Forum (n.d.) suggests:

- a deep-seated sense of meaning and purpose in life;
- a sense of belonging;
- a sense of connection of 'the deeply personal with the universal';
- acceptance, integration and a sense of wholeness.

However, spirituality is more than a notion of individuality; it involves a sense of connection with, rather than separation from, others and the world. For some people this may also entail strong connections involving place and time, 'connecting us with the living of life itself, emphasising home – a sense of place in the world – anchoring us to the land – not property, which is ephemeral – the soil that supported our ancestors now supports us' (Barker & Buchanan-Barker, 2004: xviii).

Whilst clearly for many this notion of spirituality links closely with religion, the two should not be confused or conflated. Brandon (2004) points out that although in some societies the two may be seamlessly joined, this notion of spirituality is essentially separate from organized religion and its many institutions and practices.

A social model of disability

Informed by an understanding of sociology and a social construction-ist perspective, the involvement of both theorists and activists in the disability movement has led to the development of a social model of disability, based on the view that 'Disability is something imposed on top of our impairment by the way we are unnecessarily isolated and excluded from full participation in society' (Finkelstein, 1980: 35).

Although a social model of disability owes its origins to the physical disability movement, parallels can be drawn highlighting the role of society in creating and maintaining the negative effects of mental ill health. This could be seen in the stigma and prejudice experienced by someone who talks back to their voices when walking in the street. The problem here is not the voices in themselves but the responses of others and the potential consequences of this in terms of social exclusion.

Implications for Social Work

So far in this chapter we have attempted to outline different understandings of mental health. This outline has included a brief overview of the medical model or models and their influence on understandings of mental ill health, as well as a consideration of psychological and sociological approaches and the contribution of a postmodern perspective. The influence of postmodernism on the development of diverse understandings of mental health drawing on spirituality and recovery has also been acknowledged.

We will now consider the implications of these various approaches for social workers, whether or not they see themselves as specifically practising in the mental health area. This involves considering how broader theoretical approaches can be used alongside individually created ideas of personal meaning and what this means for the reality of social work practice, as in the following example.

Practice example

Alice, a newly qualified social worker, is meeting Janice, who has been referred because she is experiencing difficulties with her young child and is depressed. Alice has a good understanding of a social perspective on mental health, having undertaken a placement in a community mental health team (CMHT). She recognizes that social isolation and poverty may be affecting Janice's mental health and is aware of the possibility that Janice may have experienced some difficulties in her own childhood.

Alice is surprised to find that Janice's understanding is based on the experience of her own mother's poor mental health, saying 'I take after my mum and she spent a long time in hospital.' In beginning to build a relationship with Janice, Alice may have to think more broadly about Janice's understanding of her own situation and how she can engage with this in order to understand and plan her work with Janice.

Alice is also concerned to make contact with the local primary mental health team, and finds that Janice could be referred for a short course of cognitive behavioural therapy (CBT) at the first tier of referral. She wonders how this will help and how this affects her own assessment of the situation. She is also aware that in the past Janice has been prescribed anti-depressant medication by her GP.

We can see from this brief example that social workers need to make sense of different paradigms and the diverse views of different professionals and agencies as well as the individual. With regard to the knowledge base, Alice will need to look at theories of health and gender as well as issues of disadvantage and social exclusion. It may also be relevant to consider issues of human development, drawing on both psychological and sociological perspectives. From the early part of this chapter, we can see that a biological or social learning model may be relevant in how Janice makes sense of her situation, whilst the prescribing of medication may indicate the influence of the medical model – or at least a professional who is hoping that this may help. Similarly the offer of CBT suggests that it is relevant to look at the contribution of a psychological perspective, specifically one that address cognitive processes and how Janice's thoughts and behaviours may be affecting her situation. What is most important here is for the worker to respect Janice's views and experiences and to use these as a basis for building a positive working relationship in which Janice is recognized as the 'expert' on her situation.

There is also the question of the extent to which social workers find themselves operating as individual practitioners in a situation such as this. How can these diverse approaches be brought together, and indeed is this helpful? The prevalence of a medical or biological model may offer less room for manoeuvre in terms of social work knowledge and skills, or offer the role of assistant when the GP asks for help in monitoring compliance with medication, or the primary mental health care team suggest that some help with child care may be valuable to enable Janice to attend for CBT. There is also the extent to which social workers working outside of specialist mental health settings and teams feel that mental health is a 'hot potato' requiring a rapid referral on to the specialist team.

Recognizing all these competing issues and questions is an important element of the process of critical reflection at the heart of social work. This requires a complex map or jigsaw of potential issues that may be relevant in any one situation and which together may begin to build up the whole picture. This could be seen as a kaleidoscope in which the various pieces and patterns form and reform depending on the particular ways they work together.

The notion of a kaleidoscope also offers the advantages of acknowledging shared or common features and experiences such as racism, sexism, homophobia or the effects of physical trauma or genetic influences, without falling into a determinist and unilinear explanation where mental ill health is attributed to just one cause. At the same time the unique sense of any individual pattern is highlighted, recognizing that no two people will have the same experience.

It is here that we return to the social meaning of mental illness and the importance of considering service users' and survivors' own understanding and meaning of their experiences. A rich and growing body of literature and other media offers access to this world and reminds us that we need to listen to these individual narratives, as the skill and the art of anyone engaging in working with people experiencing mental distress fundamentally lie in their ability to build a relationship and to engage in their world, to understand the subtleties of that unique experience, to engage in dialogue and respond in order to effect change and transformation. As has been simply stated by Parton and O'Byrne, 'It seems that telling one's story in one's own terms and having it heard respectfully is a very necessary ingredient for change to begin to occur' (2000: 12).

Concluding Comments

This chapter has offered an introduction to a broad range of thinking and perspectives on the subject of mental health and illness. Of necessity this has been brief rather than in depth, and the reader is encouraged to explore particular areas of interest further. The medical model continues to occupy a prominent position in mental health practice, yet there are a number of examples of the ways in which it has evolved in response to wider changes in thinking, prompted by the influence of mental health service users and survivors.

Alongside the medical model there is a range of psychotherapeutic, psychological and sociological perspectives, each of which offers its own particular viewpoint, and to which are now added approaches such as those emphasizing recovery and spirituality. A grasp of the many complexities involved in making sense of mental health theories and models is an essential element of mental health practice and a crucial aspect of the business of working with other practitioners and agencies.

In and amongst the various strands of this discussion, however, has been the message that social work practice benefits from the ability to draw on a range of frameworks in a flexible and sensitive fashion in order for the difficulties of any individual to be understood in an appropriate way within their own frames of reference.

Further Reading

Bracken, P. & Thomas, P. (2005) *Postpsychiatry: Mental Health in a Postmodern World*. Oxford: Oxford University Press

Read, J., Mosher, L. & Bentall, R. (eds) (2004) *Models of Madness: Psychological, Social and Biological Approaches to Schizophrenia*. Hove: Brunner Routledge

Rogers, A. & Pilgrim, D. (2000) *A Sociology of Mental Health and Illness*. 3rd edn. Maidenhead: Open University Press

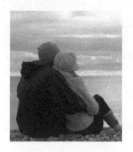

3 The Policy Framework

Key points

- The shift from institutional to community-based care
- The 'modernization' agenda and current policy drivers within health and social care
- Contemporary mental health policy
- 'Personalization' and its potential impact on mental health social work

Introduction

This chapter will begin by briefly examining the history of mental health policy in the UK in order to trace the development of current issues and developments. The wider policy drivers in health and social care and their impact on mental health will also be acknowledged, including the contradictory and contested nature of much of this landscape. Finally, the importance of policy in framing and informing mental health social work practice will be explored, recognizing some of the tensions inherent in the current emphasis on personalization.

It may be helpful to begin by considering the nature of the policy-making process, as there is a natural tendency to portray policy and legislation as the unfolding of a neat and tidy chronological process. For clarity this is reflected in the organization of this chapter. However, the reality is, by contrast, frequently confusing, contradictory and subject to conflicting ideas, interests and influences. Often the result is very different from that which was envisaged and may reflect significant changes and compromises that have taken place in order for at least some aspect of the desired changes to occur. An example of this can be found in the Mental Health Act 2007, which underwent a complex and convoluted journey, meeting with various challenges, not least the unlikely alliance of service user groups and professional bodies, before reaching the statute book. Additionally, there is often a sense that the underlying trend of legislative and policy change is positive and a manifestation of progress. Whilst this may be true in some areas – for example, the increasing recognition of human rights or user involvement in mental health care – this cannot always be assumed and there will often be a sense of 'two steps forward and one step back'. Furthermore, there may be examples of simultaneous changes in legislation or policy taking place which reflect apparently opposing interests.

The reader is therefore encouraged to keep an open mind and to consider questions such as the following:

- Whose interests were/are being served by this development?
- Who was/may be disadvantaged?
- How does this fit with the bigger picture of health and social care?
- Why is this happening now?

There is also a need to acknowledge that a text such as this can offer only a snapshot of contemporary policy at the time at which it is published, and that some aspects of this chapter will be soon be out of date. Therefore it is important that the reader keeps a close watch on more immediate sources including newspapers, professional journals and reputable internet sites.

Historical Background

Pre-industrial Britain was founded on rural life and an agrarian economy where feudal lords and the church were seen as sources of authority and protection. The main providers of care for the sick and needy were churches and monasteries, with almsgiving supporting the development of almshouses and hospitals such as St Bartholomew's, founded in 1123, St Thomas's in 1200 and Bethlem in 1247. Concerns about poverty and vagrancy in later centuries led to the creation of a national system, formalized in the Elizabethan Poor Law of 1601, which provided a range of responses for those unable to support themselves, distinguishing between those who were 'deserving' and 'undeserving' and encompassing all who did not fit in. Only in 1744 did the Vagrancy Act differentiate between vagrants and lunatics, recommending the setting up of asylums for criminal and pauper lunatics, with justices of the peace determining admissions. Care also continued to be provided in workhouses, hospitals and private madhouses at the expense of local parishes.

Although the quality of care provided was undoubtedly variable, William Battie, the first medical officer of St Luke's Hospital in London, offers an example of a pioneer in the treatment of mentally ill patients. His 1758 *Treatise on Madness* advocated the view that asylum care could be therapeutic as well as offering containment. He was followed by others such as Philippe Pinel (1745–1826), who, believing that insanity was caused by psychological factors, recommended that treatment should be firm but kind, based on good physical care and rational discussion. These ideas also influenced William Tuke, a Quaker philanthropist who opened the York Retreat for the care of the insane in 1796 on the basis of humane treatment and therapeutic occupation. Together these ideas became known as 'moral treatment'.

Despite these attempts to improve care, the beginning of the nineteenth century saw a public outcry about conditions in asylums, leading to the setting up of the Select Committee for the Better Regulation of Madhouses in England. The Committee's 1816 report (Rogers & Pilgrim, 2001: 45) describes appalling conditions of inadequate clothing and cramped and crowded accommodation with patients chained to the walls. At the same time this period saw the development of new treatments and attempts to discover the organic cause of mental illnesses, following in the footsteps of those who saw dissection as the way to developing knowledge. Such influences were increasingly to the fore as psychiatry began to achieve its own identity as a legitimate branch of medicine in the nineteenth century.

The rise of the asylums

The aftermath of the Napoleonic Wars in the early nineteenth century has been characterized as a period of growing unemployment, poverty and a high incidence of disease and malnutrition. In response, the 1834 Poor Law Amendment Act enabled the establishment of workhouses, seen as a less costly alternative to the provision of 'outdoor relief' for those unable to care for themselves and inevitably including those seen to be mentally unwell.

The 1845 Lunacy Act required the establishment of asylums in every county in England and Wales, paving the way for a system that was to last for over 100 years. Whilst influenced by the apparent success of the moral treatment pioneers, the care in the county asylums remained custodial, frequently based on physical restraint. The prevailing climate was heavily influenced by the ethos of the Poor Law and workhouse and maintained by the physical design of the buildings. These factors, together with poor conditions, an emphasis on security and staff untrained in a therapeutic approach, contributed to high mortality rates and limited chances of cure or improvement (Warner, 1994).

A number of arguments have been proposed to account for the growing numbers of people incarcerated within the county asylums, with numbers increasing by 80 per cent between the 1850s and 1900. The shift from an agricultural to a manufacturing economic base, accompanied by increasing urbanization, is seen to have played a part, whilst others point to the development of new psychiatric classification systems and the increasing professionalization of doctors (Scull, 1977). The fact that paupers remained the responsibility of the parish, whilst those seen as lunatics were transferred to the asylums, managed and financially supported by the county, may also have been relevant (Warner, 1994).

With a few notable exceptions, those outside the asylums were generally unconcerned about the plight of asylum inmates. This was reflected in the 1890 Lunacy Act, which highlighted the need to protect those outside from wrongful detention, rather than the interests of those on the inside.

Over time a number of issues began to undermine the Victorian approach to mental illness and its treatment, including growing interest in child guidance, child and family psychiatry and social psychiatry. The 1930 Mental Health Act provided for voluntary admission to hospital rather than admission through certification, with new treatments including insulin coma, ECT and leucotomy being seen to offer a sense of hope regarding the possibilities of cure and recovery. Whilst all of these remained, by and large, under the jurisdiction of the medical profession, they were supported as part of the spirit of optimism and hope that surrounded the establishment of the National Health Service (NHS) in 1948.

The decline of the asylums and the new NHS

Asylum numbers peaked in 1954 at 148,000, and this is often associated with the availability of more effective treatments, especially medication and the increasing use of major tranquillizers, enabling people to be discharged back to the community. However, Rogers and Pilgrim are sceptical of any causal link between declining numbers and a 'pharmacological revolution' (2001: 61), pointing out that this cannot account for other declining populations in institutional care such as older people or those with learning disabilities. The move towards deinstitutionalization is perhaps as likely to be linked to increasing awareness of the damaging effects of total institutions (Goffman, 1961), and as part of a wider global trend, fuelled by the growing economic costs of hospital-based care.

The 1959 Mental Health Act located new mental health services in general hospitals, a trend that was reinforced by the 1962 Hospital Plan. This move towards a greater integration of mental and physical health care can also be seen as reflecting the increasing medicalization of mental health and the growing recognition of psychiatry as a medical specialism. However, despite the renaming of asylums as hospitals, arrangements for mental health services continued to be kept separate and received significantly lower levels of funding than other areas of health care, leaving mental health, along with learning disability services, as the poor relation (Means & Smith, 1994; Lester & Glasby, 2006). Additionally, the wider infrastructure envisaged by the 1959 Act, including the provision of day centres, rehabilitation services and hostels, remained unrealized.

These changes also signified a shift of responsibility for mental health care away from local government towards the NHS, leaving the local authority with responsibilities for the compulsory admission of people to hospital and the aftercare and rehabilitation of patients. This distinction between local authority and NHS services contributed to the development of services along parallel tracks which are only now converging.

This split between health care and the local authority also has parallels in the development of mental health social work. The first training course to prepare social workers for working in mental health was set

up at the London School of Economics in 1929, following recommendations from the 1904–8 Royal Commission for the Care of the Feeble
Minded for the development of an almoner role to provide a link for
patients between home and hospital and also to support people after
their discharge. There was, however, a distinction between those
trained as psychiatric social workers, located within the hospital or
clinic setting, and the role of the Mental Welfare Officer based in the
local authority, whose responsibilities included statutory functions to
apply for compulsory admission to hospital under the 1959 Mental
Health Act. The separation of these two roles was endorsed by the
Younghusband Report (Younghusband, 1959) and only resolved by
the implementation of the Seebohm Report (1968), which created new
generic social services teams within the local authority.

Community Care

Community care can be seen as having an unsteady start in the years
from the 1960s through to the 1990s, amidst concerns that the overall
philosophy remained seriously undermined through lack of political
will, commitment and funding. There was a time lag between the
rundown of the old hospitals and the transfer of services to the new
general hospitals, and the release of funds and resources from the
old sites was slow to take place. Despite efforts at 'ring-fencing' to
ensure that resources were transferred from the institution to the community, community-based services were limited and patients on the
old long-stay wards were only gradually transferred to community-
based units.

Although attempts were made to promote and encourage joint
health and social services planning for mental health services, in
reality joint planning was piecemeal and fragile, leading to confusion
over the respective role of, for example, day centres and day hospitals
in any one area. The development of community-based mental health
teams was intended to provide support for those who had been discharged from the old long-stay hospitals, but there were concerns that
the work of the teams appeared to focus on those less in need. Social
work services, including mental health, also struggled in the face of
serious funding shortfalls for local authorities vis-à-vis the NHS, and
their increasing disfavour as providers of services within the wider
health and social care environment.

Issues of choice also remained limited as concerns about risk
remained uppermost and, despite the introduction of other safeguards, the new Mental Health Act introduced in 1983 continued to
focus on compulsory detention. The Act did bring about some changes
seen to be broadly beneficial, such as the right to advocacy for detained
patients at Mental Health Review Tribunals. Additionally, the new
Approved Social Worker role, replacing the Mental Welfare Officer of
the 1959 Act, was subject to the Mental Health Act Code of Practice,

highlighting the important contribution of a social perspective in assessment.

The lack of progress in improving services contributed to the need for a major rethink about community care in mental health as well as for older people and those with physical or learning disabilities. A major review (Griffiths, 1988) formed the basis of a report bringing together the forces of the market alongside managerialism and privatization. Accompanied by notions of choice and consumerism, these themes provided the underpinning rationale of the NHS and Community Care Act 1990. Whilst the notion of choice in care was, and remains, illusory, in terms of real choice, for those in need of mental health services, increasing recognition had to be offered both to the individual voices of patients or service users and to wider groups involved in advocacy and political campaigning on behalf of those with mental health difficulties.

The late twentieth century saw increasing claims that community care was failing, with attention focusing on a number of high-profile incidents such as the killing by Christopher Clunis of a complete stranger, Jonathan Zito, at a London Underground station. Clunis had a history of schizophrenia, and the inquiry into the case highlighted the inadequate and poorly co-ordinated care that he had received (Ritchie et al., 1994). The introduction of the Care Programme Approach in 1991 was a health initiative intended to reduce the risks of individuals falling through the net by promoting a greater co-ordination of services. However, it can also be seen to have contributed to the maintenance of a dual system, co-existing alongside local authority care management processes, each with its own paperwork. The Care Programme Approach has since been through a number of revisions and remains, in its most recent iteration, as a core element of mental health care.

Into the Twenty-First Century: The Modernization Agenda

The modernization agenda is associated with the coming to power of the 'New Labour' government in 1997, although in many ways, continuity rather than change in health and social care marked the transition from the previous Conservative government, in response to the needs of an ageing population and a volatile global economy (Fawcett & Karban, 2005). This agenda was not without its tensions, emphasizing on the one hand individual choice and the need for health and social care services to be responsive to local needs, but on the other, centralized budgets, national performance indicators and targets, and an end to the 'postcode lottery' allocation of services whereby there was considerable variation in services across the country depending on where people were living. This trend was demonstrated in the NHS Plan (Department of Health, 2000) and a series of National Service

Frameworks, each addressing a specific aspect of health, including the *National Service Framework for Mental Health* (Department of Health, 1999b), which provided an overarching policy framework for mental health setting out priorities and targets across six standards. This was complemented by the National Service Framework documents for children and young people (Department of Health, 2004c) and for older people (Department of Health, 2001b), each of which addresses the mental health needs of its respective target population.

A number of sometimes contradictory themes can be seen as crucial elements of the modernization process. These will be outlined here primarily in relation to mental health, but with some reference to the wider health and social care environment.

At one level the rhetoric of citizenship and inclusion is attractive in terms of social justice, with its emphasis on *rights and responsibilities*. Drawing on notions of social capital and strengthening communities, the use of terms such as 'choice' and 'empowerment' can, however, obscure less positive implications. For example, the emphasis on welfare to work is seen as offering inclusion and a standard of living free from dependence on state benefits as well as the wider advantages of employment. However, the implications of this for lone parents and people with mental health or other long-term health conditions are set within non-negotiable expectations and targets about the length of time that people can remain on benefits, perpetuating the stigma associated with remaining unwell or not going out to work.

The 'Third Way', associated with the same Labour government, represented an attempt to reconcile left- and right-wing policies (Giddens, 1998), seeking to bring about a compromise between the level of state control associated with 'old' Labour and the goal of privatization underpinning Conservative policies of the 1970s and 1980s. This promoted a mixed economy of care intended to create *public–private partnerships*, supported by private finance initiatives used to finance new hospitals. Increasingly this is being extended to other aspects of health and social care, such as new walk-in clinics in shopping centres, and can be seen as presenting a further threat to existing services and the role of professionals.

Inevitably, the sense of a state of perpetual reorganization has an effect on the delivery and co-ordination of services. Additionally, Local Authority Social Services Departments and Health Trusts are being required to concentrate on their commissioning role rather than service provision, which is increasingly being shifted to the private and independent sector. There is a growing private market in mental health care, including secure hospital provision, with spot purchasing for individual need, annual contracts and service level agreements.

The need for *joined-up services* to enhance effective communication and co-ordination reflects a long history of poor care highlighted by numerous inquiries and high-profile homicides, especially marked in both child protection and mental health. More generally, legislation has offered both incentive and imperative in the direction of joint commissioning and finance with the Health Act 1999 and the Health and Social Care Act 2000, although examples of complete integration of services in the form of Joint Trusts offer as yet a mixed picture in terms of success.

Whilst interprofessional and interagency working have been seen as a significant response to these challenges, there has been a concern that the agenda is simultaneously emphasizing both deprofessionalization and greater regulation as policy objectives. The latter can be seen in the Health Care Professional Act 2002 and the regulation of the social work profession. In mental health, the impetus towards changing and more flexible roles can be found in the introduction of Approved Mental Health Professionals to replace the Approved Social Worker, within the Mental Health Act 2007, and the development of new and flexible roles as demonstrated within the 'new ways of working' in mental health (Care Sector Improvement Partnership/National Institute for Mental Health in England, 2007).

A crucial aspect of the modernization agenda is an emphasis on *consumer rights* and choices and on user and carer involvement, building on the NHS and Community Care Act of 1990 and the consumerist agenda of the Conservative governments of the 1980s, and demonstrated in the Local Government and Public Involvement in Health Act 2007. Issues of equality and diversity are also highlighted with accompanying legislation to address discrimination and human rights.

Evidence-based practice is also a continuing theme in the current policy context, with an emphasis on 'what works'. Whilst there is clearly a positive strand to this, there are also considerable challenges, being informed by a predominantly quantitative research base and methodology with a clear hierarchy of evidence where service user views and feedback rate low on the scale in terms of their significance. There are also potential tensions between the form of care or treatment which is 'recommended' on the basis of the evidence and the individual choice of the service user (Frost, 2002).

A key policy driver, significantly fuelled by the rising cost of health care, can be found in the *public health* agenda. A social perspective on mental health and the current research evidence for this will be discussed in later chapters, but it is important to recognize here that the focus on mental health as a public health issue is increasingly recognized and supported by policy and guidance and offers important opportunities for social work.

Reflection point

From your understanding and experience of social work practice, can you think of any ways in which concerns about the alleged 'failure' of community care and the 'modernization agenda' have had an impact on the role and purpose of social work in mental health?

1998	*Modernising Mental Health Services*
1999	*National Service Framework for Mental Health*
1999	*Effective Care Co-ordination in Mental Health Services: Modernizing the Care Programme Approach*
2001	The journey to recovery: the Government's vision for mental health care
2002	*Women's Mental Health: Into the Mainstream*
2003	*Inside Outside: Improving Mental Health Services for Black and Minority Ethnic Communities in England*
2003	Personality Disorder – No longer a diagnosis of exclusion (policy implementation guidance for the development of services for people with personality disorder)
2004	Mental Health and Social Exclusion (Office of the Deputy Prime Minister)
2004	*The Ten Essential Shared Capabilities: A Framework for the Whole of the Mental Health Workforce*
2005	Securing Better Mental Health for Older Adults
2007	Best practice guidance: Specification for adult medium-secure services
2007	*Best Practice in Managing Risk*
2007	Capabilities for Inclusive Practice
2007	*Mental Health: New Ways of Working for Everyone*. Developing and sustaining a capable and flexible workforce. Progress Report
2008	Improving Access to Psychological Therapies Implementation Plan: National guidelines for regional delivery
2009	*New Horizons: A Shared Vision For Mental Health* (HM Government)

Figure 3.1   Summary of mental health policy 1998–2010

Contemporary Mental Health Policy

Whilst it would be impossible to review the plethora of mental health policies, reports and guidance that have been published over recent years, Figure 3.1 sets outs a time line of selected documents to convey a sense of the various aspects of this process.

New Horizons: A Shared Vision for Mental Health was launched in 2009 (Department of Health/HM Government, 2009) as a cross-government approach, bringing together national and local government, health and social services, third sector organizations, communities and individuals to promote the mental health and wellbeing of individuals and communities and to improve the quality and accessibility of services for people with mental health difficulties.

Similar policies are also in place for Northern Ireland, Wales and Scotland (Department of Health, Social Services and Public Safety, 2003; Welsh Assembly, 2005; Scottish Government, 2009). It is worth noting that whilst the strategy has generally been welcomed, its breadth and complexity may limit its overall effectiveness.

New Horizons is focused on four 'big ideas':

1. *Better mental wellbeing for individuals and communities*: to include supporting families, promoting effective parenting, environmental improvements, greater recognition of the

interrelationship between mental and physical health and increasing participation.

2. *Right help at the right time*: to offer care and treatment that is tailored to the needs of individuals and offers choice and control. Issues of access are also emphasized to ensure that disadvantaged and marginalized groups can obtain mental health and other supporting services.

3. *Improved services and access*: based on a robust evidence base regarding what works, a single comprehensive assessment, personal care packages and increasing use of technology including text messaging and telepsychiatry.

4. *Tackling discrimination*: including increased employment opportunities, addressing the portrayal of mental health in the media, anti-bullying and mental health promotion in schools and steps to address the 'double' discrimination experienced by older people or those from Black and minority ethnic communities.

Other work, such as that carried out by the Delivering Race Equality Programme, is intended to dovetail with *New Horizons* to ensure that the needs of local communities are assessed and met, that there is equality of access and outcomes with respect to services, that staff are trained in cultural competence and that inequalities are addressed (Wilson, 2009). This also emphasizes the complexity of individuals and multiple identities, and the need to respond to the unique aspects of experience, family, ethnicity, gender, age and sexuality.

Activity

Read *New Horizons: A Shared Vision for Mental Health* or the equivalent document for Scotland, Wales or Northern Ireland, and ask yourself the following questions:
- To what extent are social work and social care explicitly represented within the document?
- Could anything have been added to strengthen this?
- How hopeful are you that the aspirations contained in this are likely to result in positive changes in mental health services?

If possible find an opportunity to discuss your thoughts with others who have also read the document.

Whilst *New Horizons* is targeted at England, it is accompanied by a raft of other guidance for the whole of the UK relating to the importance of making links between employment and mental health (Health, Work and Well-Being Programme, 2009; HM Government, 2009). The introduction of mental health co-ordinators in job centres and increased links with mental health services is intended to provide support for people with mental health problems already in work and to assist others in gaining employment.

The Care Programme Approach

Introduced in 1991, and having undergone a series of revisions, the Care Programme Approach (CPA) (Department of Health, 1999a, 2008b) remains the key to the co-ordination of the assessment and planning of care for people using mental health services. The CPA is intended to apply in any situation where there is a high level of assessed risk or where care needs to be co-ordinated across a range of services, regardless of where the person is currently living. This in effect crosses the boundaries between hospital, supported accommodation, independent living and, where relevant, prison.

A central principle of the CPA is that the service user remains at the heart of the assessment and planning process, which also emphasizes social inclusion and recovery, paying attention to all aspects of the person's life, including their family and social relationships, housing and occupation, spirituality and overall mental and physical wellbeing as well as issues of risk. The role of the Care Co-ordinator is key to ensuring that the care plan is implemented and regularly reviewed, with changes being made in response to changing needs or circumstances. Care plans also need to include a contingency or crisis plan with reference to Advanced Statements where these have been made to enable users to set out how they want to be treated.

Service users' experiences of the CPA have been mixed in terms of their level of involvement and control over the process. Effective relationships between the service user, carers and Care Co-ordinator are central to the success of the process, with guidance referring to 'therapeutic partnerships' supported by trust and long-term engagement. The involvement of service users at every level includes being involved in decisions as to where and when CPA meetings should take place and who should attend, rather than these solely being required to fit organizational demands or the diaries of practitioners. Carers are also viewed as playing an essential part in the CPA, recognizing their contribution to care as well as their own needs for support.

Carers

Carers have increasingly been recognized within policy since their formal acknowledgement within the NHS and Community Care Act 1990, although reports (Pinfold & Corry, 2003b) continue to emphasize that their experiences and needs remain invisible and unheard. Standard 6 of the *National Service Framework* (Department of Health, 1999b) offered all those providing regular and substantial care for a person on the CPA an annual assessment and their own written care plan, although there is only limited evidence regarding the successful meeting of this target. The *New Horizons* document, despite referring to carers as a 'vital resource' (Department of Health/HM Government, 2009: 59) requiring information and possible support, pays less detailed attention to how these needs might be met. although it does refer to the government's ten-year strategy, *Carers at the Heart of 21st Century Families and Communities*, which offers a number of recommendations. This sets out that by 2018:

- carers will be respected as expert care partners and will have access to the integrated and personalised services they need to support them in their caring role;
- carers will be able to have a life of their own alongside their caring role;
- carers will be supported so that they are not forced into financial hardship by their caring role;
- carers will be supported to stay mentally and physically well and treated with dignity;
- children and young people will be protected from inappropriate caring and have the support they need to learn, develop and thrive, to enjoy positive childhoods and to achieve against all the *Every Child Matters* [Department for Education and Skills, 2004] outcomes.   (HM Government, 2008: 16)

Information about the numbers of people involved in providing care in general, taken from the 2001 census, indicates that there are 5.67 million carers in Britain, of whom 58 per cent are women (Department of Health, 2009b: 4). The demands of caring and the implications for carers' own mental health are also recognized, with those providing care for someone in the same household having significantly worse mental health, particularly those caring for a partner or a child. One in three carers surveyed found that their social relationships and leisure activities were adversely affected, and 9 per cent were taking anti-depressants, sedatives or sleeping tablets (Singleton et al., 2000). Within the bigger picture of independent living and the personalization agenda, it would appear that the role of carers and the associated personal demands and stressors can only become increasingly significant.

Within mental health it is recognized that informal carers play an essential role in providing support to adults experiencing mental health difficulties (Department of Health, 2002c), with an estimated 1.5 million caring for someone with a mental illness or dementia (Rethink, 2006). A survey of mental health carers carried out in 2003 (Pinfold & Corry, 2003a) found that 41 per cent of respondents stated that their mental and physical health had been affected, with 60 per cent saying that being a carer had an impact on their life outside the home; 89 per cent had significant health needs of their own. Only one in five had received a carer's assessment and of these only a half felt that their needs had been met.

Reflection point

Consider any potential tensions in involving carers in the CPA.
How could social workers and teams work best to resolve these?

Personalization and Mental Health Social Work Practice

Personalization has been defined as: 'People with mental health needs having choice and control over their care with support and resources provided by the local authority' (Mind, 2009: 3). The concept is seen to include a range of different initiatives including direct payments, individual budgets and personal budgets, all of which are further defined in Figure 3.2.

The personalization agenda has been seen as representing both a logical next step in a constantly evolving process of policy development and a paradigm shift in thinking about care. In terms of the former, the origins of personalization can be found in the increasing attention being paid to the voices of service users and carers, drawing particularly from the physical disability movement, growing emphasis on choice and involvement and the move towards recovery and social inclusion for people with mental health difficulties. At the same time, the shift away from institutional care, service-led assessments and professional expertise, and towards an ethos of rights and citizenship and the **co-production** of care, demonstrates a potentially transformative step-change in the way in which care and support are offered and accessed.

Choice and control are seen to be integral to the meaning and the practice of personalization as well as essential in reinforcing social inclusion. Advocates of personalization point to the 'fit' with social work values and approaches to practice based on service users' strengths and resources, suggesting that it offers new possibilities for social work by (re)claiming a leadership role in determining the future development of mental health services and influencing practice from a social perspective embedded in values of social justice (Ray et al., 2008; Allen et al., 2009).

Co-production a term increasingly used in health and social care to describe how the responsibility for health and wellbeing is shared between health and social care agencies and the individual.

- *Personal budget*: An individual allocation of social care money which can be used to purchase support and care, possibly from existing services and without necessarily involving money being paid to the service user.

- *Individual budget*: Similar to a personal budget but potentially drawing on funds from other funding streams such as Supporting People or the Independent Living Fund.

- *Direct payments*: Cash payments paid directly to service users to enable them to buy their own support.

Figure 3.2 Terms associated with personalization
Source: Adapted from Mind (2009)

A note of scepticism has been raised, however, in response to these claims. In particular, attention has been drawn to the limitations of personalization in promoting social inclusion for people with learning disabilities, especially within the current context of global economic downturn (Boxall et al., 2009; Radley, 2009). The dichotomy of professionalization and personalization in relation to the co-production of health and the employment of health trainers has also been challenged (Lhussier & Carr, 2008). Ferguson (2007: 388) addresses the 'multiple meanings' and 'overwhelmingly positive' nature of much of the debate surrounding personalization, suggesting that the attraction rests within the inherent ambiguity of the concept, in appearing to reject paternalism whilst simultaneously being entirely in line with the themes of individual choice and responsibility and the privatization of risk at the heart of welfare reform. He argues that this takes place without reference to the need to address fundamental social inequalities which impact on those groups and individuals who are most likely to use social work and mental health services, and whose lives are likely to offer fewer choices and potentially greater risks, including that of being subject to the more coercive aspects of care and treatment, such as the compulsory powers of the mental health legislation.

Ferguson also draws attention to the potential for personalization to act as a smokescreen for cost-cutting and reduction in provision whilst increasing the opportunities for the privatization of services. Responding to those who suggest that personalization offers new opportunities to reinvigorate social work, there is also the suggestion that personalization can only contribute to the deprofessionalization and deskilling of the profession. As an alternative Ferguson proposes that social work needs to 'develop and strengthen *collective* organisation amongst those who use services and amongst those who provide them' (Ferguson, 2007: 401).

In concluding this discussion we need to recognize the uncertain and contested nature of the personalization debate and attempt to avoid any simplistic or neat conclusions. It may be that in different times and places personalization may offer positive opportunities for individual choice and access to resources or activities that will promote wellbeing, recovery and social inclusion. At other times and in other contexts, social workers and service users may need to work together to challenge the rhetoric of choice that may obscure reductions in the provision of care or the maintenance of systems and processes that perpetuate inequalities. Strategies of this kind require vigilance and close attention to an agenda of promoting social justice that lies at the heart of social work practice.

Concluding Comments

The policy context for mental health is complex and multifaceted, influenced by a number of dynamic and sometimes contradictory themes. In particular, there are issues relating to the way in which mental health and illness are understood and the various discourses that accompany this in terms of medical and social models, risk and recovery, and social inclusion. These are also located within the wider reform agenda for health and social care including concerns regarding the power of professionals, such as social workers, and the growing financial costs of provision against a backdrop of global economic downturn.

For social workers attempting to navigate this terrain, the way can appear fraught with difficulty and uncertainty. This chapter does not offer any easy solutions, but has attempted to set out the framework within which practice takes place and to introduce some of the tensions and conflicting demands that may arise. The discussion reinforces the need for critical reflection and living with uncertainty that, for many, characterizes social work, and emphasizes the need to ground practice in social work values and ethics.

Further Reading

Lester, H. & Glasby, J. (2006) *Mental Health Policy and Practice.* Basingstoke: Palgrave Macmillan

Rogers, A. & Pilgrim, D. (2001) *Mental Health Policy in Britain.* 2nd edn. Basingstoke: Palgrave Macmillan

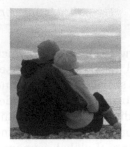

4 The Legal Framework

Key points

- The origins and development of key legislation relating to mental health including the Mental Health 2007
- The relationship between the Mental Health Act and the Mental Incapacity Act 2005
- Tensions within the current legislative framework and the balance between issues of risk and dangerousness versus recovery and social justice
- The relevance of the wider legislative and policy context for social work practice

Introduction

The chapter will consider some of the key issues relating to mental health legislation in England and Wales, with brief reference to the wider context of the United Kingdom. New roles including the Approved Mental Health Professional and the Responsible Clinician will be introduced and their implications for social work explored. Additionally, links will be made to other relevant areas of legislation including the Mental Capacity and Community Care Acts and human rights legislation. Finally, the importance of legislation and policy in framing and informing mental health social work practice will be explored.

Current Legislation

The legislation surrounding mental health is detailed and complex and can appear bewildering to service users and their carers as well as to social workers and other professionals. Simply keeping pace with changes and new case law can be very demanding and it is likely that things will change and develop, even between the completion of a text such as this and its reaching the shelves of a library or book shop. For these reasons, this part of the chapter will address the key points and significant issues and their implications for social work practice, whilst recommending that current and reputable resources are consulted when precise information is required. This is requisite for social work practice in any field, embedded as it is within legislation and policy frameworks: when working with people experiencing mental health difficulties there are also especially significant issues relating to compulsory detention, treatment and rights. For those social workers who undertake further training to become an Approved Mental Health Professional, a detailed knowledge of and familiarity with the law are essential.

Before considering the legislation that specifically applies to mental health, it is important to consider relevant aspects of the broader legislative context that also play an important part.

Activity

Think about the general legislation that is relevant for social work practice. Draw up a list and note the reasons why this is relevant to mental health. Compare your list with the one in Figure 4.1.

Figure 4.1 excludes legislation that specifically relates to mental health as this will be considered separately. Do not be surprised if you have some additional points in your 'Activity' list, as there are many relevant areas that could be included.

Much of this legislation relates to civil liberties and human rights and it is evident that there are many areas where people who have experienced mental health difficulties have been discriminated against. For example, the 1974 Juries Act prohibits anyone from serving on a jury who has 'mental illness, psychopathic disorder, mental handicap or severe mental handicap, and on account of that condition either is resident in a hospital or other similar institution, or regularly attends for treatment by a medical practitioner'. Whilst it is recognized that legislation such as this is outdated, at the time of writing this still stands and is currently the subject of campaigning and action to amend the law in line with the Mental Capacity Act (Rethink, 2010).

Human rights and equalities legislation

The Human Rights Act 1998 has been seen as key to protecting civil liberties in respect of mental health, and certain articles are especially relevant. These include:

- *Article 2*: protects right to life, which may be relevant in terms of negligence or leaving people at risk of suicide;
- *Article 3*: prohibits torture, inhuman or degrading treatment, which may include mistreatment although not the side effects of prescribed medication;
- *Article 5*: protects right to liberty and security, which can only be removed if professional judgement provides justification on grounds of the nature or severity of disorder and must be subject to safeguards;

Date	Legislation	Provisions
1984	Police and Criminal Evidence Act	Includes provision for detention, treatment and questioning and the involvement of an 'appropriate adult' where required
1990	NHS and Community Care Act	Provides overall framework for community care including mental health
1995	Disability Discrimination Act	Makes it illegal to discriminate against people with a disability on certain grounds
1995	Carers (Recognition and Services) Act	Provides carers with rights to assessment, subject to some limitations
1998	Human Rights Act	Upholds the European Convention on Human Rights
2000	Data Protection Act	Enables access to health, housing and social services records
2000	Carers and Disabled Children Act	Strengthens rights of carers over 16 years of age to an assessment
2002	Nationality, Immigration and Asylum Act	Amends support arrangements for asylum seekers and creates provisions for detention and removal
2003	Anti-Social Behaviour Act	Extends provision of anti-social behaviour orders in UK (first introduced in Crime and Disorder Act 1998)
2004	Domestic Violence, Crime and Victims Act	Extends provision to combat domestic violence
2004	Carers (Equal Opportunities) Act	Ensures that carers are informed of rights to assessment and that their outside interests are recognized
2004	Children Act	Relates to safeguarding of children, including a duty to co-operate between services and creation of Local Safeguarding Children Boards. Also creates electronic records for all children
2005	Disability Discrimination Act	Creates a legal duty for public authorities to promote disability equality
2010	Equality Act	Brings together and streamlines discrimination legislation across all areas

Figure 4.1   Broader legislation relevant for mental health practice

- *Article 8*: protects right to privacy, family life and home, which can be interpreted as relating to the adequate provision of support in order to enable someone to remain at home and also to issues of contact with relatives and hospital visits etc.

Many of these rights are in fact qualified and open to interpretation. However, the legislation does offer a means of challenging unfair treatment.

Whilst the Disability Discrimination Acts of 1995 and 2005, and a number of related amendments, have also been viewed as significant in offering protection from discrimination on the grounds of mental health, this has now been brought together in the Equality Act 2010, which incorporates a broad range of legislation relating to race, sex, age, disability, sexual orientation, religion and belief. This states that a 'disabled' person is someone with 'a physical or mental impairment which has a substantial and long-term adverse effect on his/her ability to carry out normal day-to-day activities' (Equality Act 2010, Section 6). Such a definition will include many people experiencing mental health difficulties and has been seen as offering protection against a range of areas in which discrimination on the grounds of mental ill health has taken place.

Reflection point

Think of an example from practice where human rights and equalities legislation would be relevant in challenging discrimination. What additional knowledge and skills might you need in order to develop your practice in this area?

Mental Health Acts 1983 and 2007

Current legislation in England and Wales is determined by the Mental Health Act 1983 as amended by the Mental Health Act 2007. The need for new legislation was identified as part of the 'modernizing' approach to mental health services (Department of Health, 1998) and to a large extent was driven by a political agenda focused on issues of risk and dangerousness. This included concerns regarding the availability and provision of treatment for people with personality disorders following in the wake of several high-profile cases. Additionally there was seen to be a need to provide compulsory treatment in the community to address the problem of people discontinuing treatment and becoming unwell after they had left hospital.

The journey to new legislation, however, was not straightforward, and various unsuccessful attempts were made before the new Act was agreed. Of particular significance was the development of an alliance between service user and professional organizations united in their opposition to the various proposals. In addition to concerns regarding the introduction of compulsory treatment in the community, other areas included the implications of the replacement of the role of the Approved Social Worker with that of the **Approved Mental Health Professional (AMHP)**. More positively, the new legislation updated the definition of the nearest relative to include civil partners, introduced new treatment safeguards and provided for access to independent advocates for detained patients. There is also provision for age-appropriate services for children and young people.

Approved Mental Health Professional (AMHP) a qualified social worker, mental health nurse, occupational therapist or psychologist who has undergone additional training approved by the General Social Care Council and been approved to undertake duties under the Mental Health Act. (The Mental Health (Approved Mental Health Professionals) (Approval) (England) Regulations 2008 No. 1206)

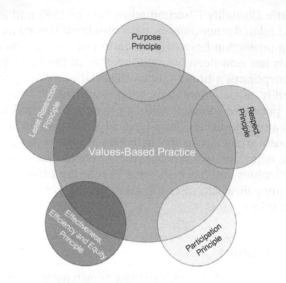

Figure 4.2 Mental Health Act guiding principles
Source: King et al. (n.d.)

A number of the key areas of the provision of the mental health legislation will be broadly outlined here, although readers are advised to refer to more detailed law texts and the Acts themselves, as well as the accompanying *Code of Practice* (Department of Health, 2008a), for accurate and current information. The *Code of Practice* is generally recognized as providing advice on how to implement the Act in general, supported by the guiding principles which are seen to assist in applying the Act in individual situations (see Figure 4.2).

Definition of mental disorder

The 2007 Act modified the definition of mental disorder as 'any disorder or disability of mind'. This definition does not include learning disability unless this is associated with abnormally aggressive or seriously irresponsible conduct. In all cases, for the longer-term powers of detention, an appropriate medical treatment test must be satisfied. This provision was introduced to avoid the situation whereby certain potential patients were not admitted to hospital on the grounds that they were not 'treatable'. The *Code of Practice* (E para. 6.7) states that this is to ensure that no one is detained unless they are actually to be offered medical treatment, although there are no guarantees required that the treatment will be effective, simply that it is available. Additionally, the definition of treatment is broad, encompassing the spectrum of approaches within a broadly therapeutic approach, rather than specific forms of medication or therapy.

Civil sections for compulsory admission (Part 2)

The process of compulsory admission involves two doctors, one of whom must be a Section 12 approved doctor with special experience in the diagnosis and treatment of mental disorder. Both doctors must agree that the person needs to be in hospital and are willing to recommend detention. It is generally recommended that at least one of the doctors should have previous knowledge of the patient. An AMHP then decides whether or not to make an application for the person's compulsory admission to hospital. In doing so the AMHP must satisfy themselves that the relevant legal criteria are met and that any application is made with regard to any wishes of the patient or their family and to any special circumstances. The role of the AMHP requires that they must interview the person 'in a suitable manner' and must consider the least restrictive options and alternatives to hospital, as well as issues of language and culture. It is also possible for the nearest relative to make an application in the place of the AMHP, although this is unusual.

Section 2

Under Section 2, it must be determined that the person is suffering from a mental disorder and needs to be detained for assessment (or assessment followed by medical treatment) for their own health or safety, or the protection of others. This section lasts for up to twenty-eight days. It cannot be renewed, but the person may be assessed for Section 3 before the twenty-eight days expire.

Section 3

The criteria for Section 3 are that the person has a mental disorder, and that admission to hospital is necessary for their own health or safety or the protection of others, and treatment cannot be provided unless they are detained in hospital. Section 3 can last for up to six months and is renewable, initially for six months and then on a yearly basis.

Section 4

In an emergency, where the criteria for Section 2 are met but there is no time to wait for a second medical recommendation, it is possible to admit someone under Section 4 with only one medical recommendation in support of an application. The second medical recommendation must be obtained within seventy-two hours.

Nearest Relative

The nearest relative is clearly defined within the legislation, and it is the role of the AMHP to determine who this is. In addition, the AMHP is required to inform or consult the nearest relative when a Section 2 or 3 is being considered. In the case of a Section 3, the nearest relative has the power to object to the application, which cannot then proceed unless the AMHP takes steps to have the nearest relative displaced by the county court on the grounds that they are objecting unreasonably. The Act also provides for the patient to displace their own nearest relative in court on the grounds that they are 'unsuitable'. The nearest relative can also take steps to authorize someone else to carry out this function if they do not feel that this role is appropriate or feasible.

The following list is used to determine the nearest relative:

- husband or wife or civil partner (or living as such for a minimum of six months);
- son or daughter;
- father or mother;
- brother or sister;
- grandparent;
- grandchild;
- uncle or aunt;
- nephew or niece;
- any other person with whom the patient has resided for five years or more.

If more than one person is identified, the person nearest the top of the list is the nearest relative, with precedence given to the elder of any two in one category and to full-blood rather than half-blood relationships.

The 'Practice example' illustrates some of the various aspects of a compulsory admission to hospital, including the role of the AMHP in making the application and contacting the nearest relative. In reality the process of co-ordinating an assessment and admission is even more highly complex and demanding of the AMHP than this example might suggest.

Practice example

Marie is a social worker based in a Community Mental Health Team and is also an AMHP. Whilst on duty she receives a referral regarding a 25-year-old man. Stephen is unemployed and lives on his own in a bedsit. He has a brother, Paul, who has become concerned about Stephen as he appears not to be going to bed, and spends most of his time watching the television. Some nights Paul has received over twenty incoherent text messages from Stephen, referring to how he is being watched and how the television is communicating directly with him. On a recent visit Stephen was initially reluctant to let Paul into his bedsit and told him that he had a carving knife and an iron bar hidden under the sofa to protect himself.

Marie agrees that there are clearly some issues of concern, but decides to see initially if she can find out any information about Stephen's history. She talks to Stephen's GP, who is not aware of any history of mental health difficulties, and also contacts Paul, as it would appear that he is the person most in contact with Stephen at present. Paul informs her that he has tried to suggest that Stephen gets some help but that he has refused. Marie also alerts the consultant in the team and contacts the police due to concerns about the possibility of Stephen becoming violent, although she recognizes that the presence of the police can potentially inflame the situation.

On meeting with Stephen, the consultant, who is a Section 12 doctor, and Stephen's GP are both of the opinion that Stephen has a mental disorder and needs further assessment as an inpatient. Attempts to discuss an informal hospital admission are met with resistance from Stephen. Marie, however, needs to make her own independent decision about whether an application for compulsory admission to hospital is appropriate. She considers whether or not the Crisis Resolution and Home Treatment Team might be able to offer sufficient support for Stephen at home, in keeping with the principle of the 'least restrictive alternative', but she remains anxious about his safety and that of others, including his brother, as Stephen appears very distressed about the people talking to him through the television. He claims they are threatening to harm him and that they are some old friends of his that live nearby. Marie is also aware of the risks associated with a compulsory hospital admission, including the consequences of Stephen being seen to be taken away by police car or ambulance, as well as the impact in terms of his civil and human rights and future employment. On balance she decides that a compulsory admission is justifiable on the grounds of Stephen's potential threat to others as well as the need to avoid a further deterioration in his mental health.

The decision is made to admit Stephen under Section 2 of the Mental Health Act, which provides for assessment and treatment, lasts for twenty-eight days and is often seen to be most appropriate when someone is not already known to the mental health services. Unlike Section 3, under which Marie would have to consult with the nearest relative, whose agreement would be required, Section 2 requires that the nearest relative simply be informed. Although Stephen's brother has been closely involved with the situation, it is in fact Stephen's father who is the nearest relative, as Stephen does not have a wife or civil partner, or anyone with whom he has been living as a partner, or any children. His mother is no longer alive and his father is therefore the person nearest the top of the list.

Marie makes sure that she contacts Stephen's father and informs him and Paul about the implications of a compulsory hospital admission. She follows the police car that takes Stephen to the hospital and makes sure that the paperwork is complete and correct, as well as checking that Stephen will be given the necessary information about his rights.

Section 5

Section 5 gives the power of detaining someone who is already an informal patient in hospital. A psychiatric nurse can hold someone for up to six hours (S5.4) and a doctor can hold someone for up to seventy-two hours (S5.2), to allow time for an assessment to take place. The person must be seen to be suffering from a mental disorder, and detention must be seen to be justified in order to safeguard their health and safety or the protection of others.

Section 7: Guardianship

An application to the local authority for guardianship can be made under Section 7 if someone is suffering from a mental disorder and it is necessary in the interests of their welfare or the protection of others that they should receive care within the community which they would otherwise refuse. A guardianship order requires two medical recommendations and an application from an AMHP or the nearest relative, and a named guardian is required, usually the local services department. The requirements of the section concern a specific place of residence and attendance at specific times and places for treatment, occupation or training, and also allows access to a doctor, AMHP or other specified person.

Guardianship has not been widely used as it is not seen to offer compulsion if the person refuses to co-operate, raising the paradoxical situation that it will only work where the individual agrees to the requirements of the order. However, there are situations where guardianship has been seen to be helpful in implementing care plans. It is worth noting that guardianship is not seen as a means of depriving someone of their liberty, although the development of case law in relation to both the Mental Capacity Act and the Mental Health Act may lead to changes in how this is understood.

Responsible Clinician a role, created by the Mental Health Act 2007, with overall responsibility for a patient's care. Previously this responsibility rested with the Responsible Medical Officer, who was required to be a medical doctor. Responsible Clinicians play a part in making, varying or discharging Community Treatment Orders, can discharge patients from detention or guardianship, and generally play an important role in ensuring that patients' needs are met.

Section 17A: Supervised Community Treatment

Section 17A allows certain patients to be discharged from hospital subject to being recalled if necessary to receive compulsory treatment. Despite fears that this might lead to situations where nurses might be expected to administer medication against someone's will in their own home, this is not the case, and treatment cannot be enforced in the community.

Supervised Community Treatment (SCT), also known as Community Treatment Orders, can be applied to patients liable to be detained under Section 3 / 37 and Part 3 unrestricted patients (see 'Court Sections (Part 3)' below) where the **Responsible Clinician** and the AMHP agree that mental disorder as defined by the Act is present, that appropriate treatment is available and necessary for the health and safety of the patient or others and that treatment can be provided without continued detention in hospital.

As yet there is only limited information available as to the use of SCT. Evidence from New Zealand (Mullen et al., 2006), where similar legislation exists, suggests that some family members, whilst mindful of the ethical considerations involved, have found the provision reassuring in that it provides back-up and influence on the care of the individual concerned, and can be seen to have benefits in terms of the outcomes. Early findings of the Mental Health Act Commission (2009) suggest that the numbers of people subject to SCT in the first six months of the implementation of the Act were higher than expected and that Black Caribbean patients, already over-represented in the detained population, could be even more disproportionately represented within this group. Concerns are also raised regarding the potential for SCT to be the default option when detained patients are discharged, with the report pointing to the increase in conditional discharge arrangements for restricted patients under Part 3 of the Act.

Other powers

The Act also provides other powers to enable the assessment of people in the community. Section 135 enables an AMHP to obtain a warrant to enter someone's home if they are living alone and not caring for themselves, or if there are concerns that someone is being cared for by someone else but not being kept 'under proper care or control'. Section 136 provides the police with powers to remove someone who appears to be suffering from a mental disorder, and who is in need of care or control, from a public place to a place of safety, in order for an assessment to be carried out. Within this definition a 'place of safety' may include police cells or a psychiatric intensive care unit (PICU). The Thirteenth Biennial Report of the Mental Health Act Commission (2009) points out that this remains the only example of a civil power to detain a patient that does not require a statutory form. Particular concern is expressed regarding the lack of adequate data regarding its use, especially in relation to ethnic monitoring in the light of information that suggests that people from Black and minority ethnic groups are over-represented.

Court sections (Part 3)

A separate range of provisions is in place under Part 3 of the Mental Health Act relating to mentally disordered offenders. It is important to note that the nearest relative plays only a limited role in this part of the Act and that anyone detained under a hospital order is not eligible to apply to the Mental Health Review Tribunal within the first six months.

The presence of any mental disorder and its likely impact on any criminal proceedings will also be considered by the Crown Prosecution Service in its decision-making regarding prosecution. Sections 35, 36 and 48 (see below) apply before the person is tried in court, with other sections being applied at the point of conviction or sentencing.

Section 35

Section 35 provides for remand to hospital for reports for a maximum of twelve weeks. This requires either the magistrates or the Crown Court to have evidence from one doctor that the person has a mental disorder, and that it would be impractical for a report to be made if they were given bail.

Section 36

Section 36 enables remand to hospital for treatment for a maximum of twelve weeks. This section can only be made by the Crown Court and requires the evidence of two doctors that the person is suffering from a mental disorder of a nature or degree that makes remand to hospital for treatment appropriate.

Section 48

Section 48 allows for two doctors to agree that a remand prisoner be urgently admitted to hospital for medical treatment, on the grounds that the person is suffering from a mental disorder of a nature or degree which makes such an admission to hospital for the purpose of medical treatment appropriate.

Section 37: hospital order

A hospital order can be made by the Crown Court and requires evidence from two registered medical practitioners that a person is suffering from a mental disorder and that a hospital order is the most appropriate disposal. This lasts for six months and is then renewable in the first instance for a further six months and then yearly. If it is renewed, the person can apply to a Mental Health Review Tribunal. The order can be discharged by the Responsible Clinician. The Crown Court also has the power to impose a term of imprisonment, but with a direction that the person be transferred to hospital for immediate treatment (Section 45A).

Section 38

Section 38 allows for assessment and compulsory treatment following conviction for an imprisonable offence (except murder) where the court wishes to reserve the final decision on sentencing until such time as it is clear that treatment is appropriate. This order is initially made for twelve weeks and is then renewable for up to twenty-eight days at a time, to a maximum of one year, after which the Court will pass its final sentence, which may be a Section 37 hospital order.

Section 41: restriction order

In serious cases, a restriction order may be made 'without limit of time' to protect the public from serious harm. Only the Secretary of State from the Ministry of Justice has the power to grant leave, transfer or discharge.

Section 47

Under Section 47, after sentencing, a prisoner can be transferred from prison to psychiatric hospital if two doctors agree that the person is suffering from a mental disorder requiring detention in hospital for treatment and that appropriate treatment is available. Such a transfer is similar to a Section 37 hospital order and may also be accompanied by a restriction order. Any restriction order will end at the expiry of the original sentence.

Treatment (Part 4)

The 2007 Mental Health Act offers new safeguards in electroconvulsive therapy (ECT), in addition to the consent-to-treatment provisions contained within Part 4 of the 1983 Act. Consent to medical treatment should always be sought. Part 4 states that treatment for mental disorder can be given *without* consent if a person is detained under Sections 2, 3, 36, 37, 38, 45A, 47 or 48. Patients on SCT are subject to Part 4 of the Act at times when they are recalled to hospital. Other 'emergency' sections of the act, such as 4, 5 and 136, do not allow for treatment without consent.

A key role here is that of the Second Opinion Appointed Doctor (SOAD), who acts on behalf of the Mental Health Act Commission to provide an independent opinion. This applies when psychiatric medication has been given to a patient for three months without consent and a decision is required as to whether or not this should continue (Section 58/A).

ECT cannot be given without the patient's consent unless they are assessed as being not capable of understanding its nature, purpose and likely effects, and a SOAD agrees that it is appropriate. In addition ECT cannot be given if a valid advance decision has been made by the patient refusing ECT, regardless of their ability to understand its nature, purpose and likely effects at the time that the treatment is being proposed. Similarly, ECT cannot be given if this conflicts with a decision of an attorney appointed under a Lasting Power of Attorney, or of a deputy appointed by the Court of Protection or by the Court itself. Section 62 of the Act does permit ECT to be given without consent in an emergency, even if the patient is capable of understanding the treatment.

In situations where psychosurgery is being considered for either formal or informal patients, Section 57 states that treatment cannot be given without informed consent and a second opinion confirming that it is appropriate.

Advocacy, tribunals and appeals

The Act created the role of the Independent Mental Health Advocate (IMHA) for those patients who are either detained or subject to Community Treatment Orders or guardianship. Advocacy is seen to provide help in accessing relevant information about the Mental Health Act in respect of the patient's circumstances, their care and treatment and their rights and access to representation.

Mental Health Review Tribunals have the power to review cases of detained patients and to consider whether they should remain under section, and the power to order direct discharge if appropriate. The tribunal consists of three members (a legal, a medical and a lay representative), and in each case, the burden of proof is on those arguing for continued detention. The legal representative acts as the chair of the tribunal and the medical member of the tribunal will also examine the patient in advance of the hearing.

Patients detained under Section 2 are able to apply to the tribunal in the first fourteen days of their detention, and those under Section 3 or guardianship may apply once in the initial six months of their detention and once thereafter within each renewal period, with similar provision for those patients subject to Community Treatment Orders.

Hospital managers also have responsibilities to ensure that patients are referred to the Mental Health Review Tribunal if they have not already applied themselves. In the case of patients under Section 3 of the Act, this is within six months of their first detention.

Until 2009, responsibility for the overall scrutiny of the Mental Health Act, including the safeguarding of the interests of those detained, rested with the Mental Health Act Commission (MHAC), whose reports were widely recognized and respected. This responsibility now rests with the Care Quality Commission, which appoints independent Mental Health Act Commissioners and SOADs as well as undertaking the other functions previously associated with the MHAC.

Mental Capacity Act 2005

The Mental Capacity Act 2005 provides a legal framework for people over the age of 16 who are seen to lack capacity in relation to the handling of everyday health, care and treatment as well as financial matters and legal affairs. The Act is also closely related to the Mental Health Act 2007, which provided amendments to authorize the deprivation of liberty of a person in a hospital or care home who lacks capacity to consent to being there. Known as the 'Deprivation of Liberty Safeguards' (DoLS), these were introduced in response to the 2004 Bournewood judgement and European Court of Human Rights ruling.

The Bournewood case concerned a man with autism whose behaviour caused concern whilst he was attending a day centre and who was subsequently admitted to hospital for three months. During this time contact with his carers was restricted and they were also unable to discharge him. Although he did not resist or refuse treatment, it was later determined in the European Court of Human Rights (*HL* v. *UK* 2004) that he lacked capacity to consent to hospital admission and treatment and that his liberty was restricted in a number of ways.

The DoLS allow for the deprivation of liberty of a person in a care home or hospital following an assessment by a **Best Interest Assessor (BIA)** together with a Section 12 approved doctor or one with a minimum of three years post-registration experience.

In relation to assessing capacity, Section 2 of the 2005 Act states that: 'a person lacks capacity in relation to a matter if at the material time he is unable to make a decision for himself in relation to the matter because of an impairment of, or a disturbance in the functioning of, the mind or brain'. A person is unable to make a decision if they are unable to do one or more of the following things, set out in Section 3 of the Act:

- understand the information relevant to the decision;
- retain the information for long enough to be able to make a decision;
- use or weigh up the information as part of the process of making the decision;
- communicate the decision by any possible method, such as talking, using sign language, squeezing someone's hand and so on.

> **Best Interest Assessor (BIA)** an AMHP, social worker, nurse, occupational therapist or psychologist with two years post-qualifying experience who has successfully completed approved BIA training. Their role is to determine whether or not someone lacks capacity and, if they do, whether or not, and how, it is appropriate to restrict their liberty.

It is essential that the Act is considered in the light of the accompanying *Code of Practice* (Department for Constitutional Affairs, 2007), which contains the guiding principles set out below:

1. A person must be assumed to have capacity unless it is established they do not.
2. A person is not to be treated as unable to make a decision unless all practicable steps have been taken to help them.
3. A person is not to be treated as unable to make a decision because they make an unwise decision.
4. Any act or decision made on behalf of someone must be in their best interests.
5. Least restrictive option must always be considered.

(Office of the Public Guardian, 2009: 13)

Additionally, it is emphasized that capacity can only be determined at a particular time in relation to a particular decision. It is not enough that someone has a particular condition or diagnosis or has experienced certain symptoms that might, on occasions, limit their capacity to make decisions.

The Act also provides for planning for future loss of capacity by enabling people to make Advance Decisions or a Lasting Power of

Attorney. Advance decisions concern the refusal of treatment and can be made by capacitated adults. They need not be in writing unless life-sustaining treatment is being considered, and must state what treatment cannot be given and under what circumstances. Advance Decisions can be over-ridden if Part 4 of the Mental Health Act applies. Lasting Powers of Attorney (LPA) contain prescribed information and must be witnessed and registered. They can be made by capacitated adults and relate to personal welfare matters and/or property and legal affairs, allowing the appointment of an attorney to make decisions on the person's behalf if they no longer have the capacity.

In cases where advance plans have not been made, the Court of Protection (Mental Capacity Act 2005, Section 45(1)) can make decisions on behalf of an incapacitated person on a wide range of matters including personal welfare, medical decision issues and property.

Mental Health Legislation across the United Kingdom

It is beyond the scope of this book to address the detail of mental health legislation outside of England and Wales, and it is worth noting that even for Wales, there are some differences in the accompanying regulations of the Mental Health Act, as well as different paperwork and a separate Code of Practice. There are interesting comparisons to be made, however, in terms of the different legislation. For example, it has been suggested that, unlike England, where there has been a greater emphasis on public safety, in Scotland, issues of safeguarding patients' rights are a major priority (Szmukler & Holloway, 2000; Hothersall et al., 2008).

Mental health law in Scotland was altered in 2003, following the recommendations of the Millan Committee (Scottish Executive, 2001). The resulting Mental Health (Care and Treatment) (Scotland) Act 2003 is based on ten principles and emphasizes compulsory treatment rather than hospitalization, with a new, community-based compulsory treatment order to replace the previous long-term hospital order. Unlike in England and Wales, the role of the Mental Health Officer remains solely within the social work profession, and they alone can consent to most emergency and all short-term detentions and apply for compulsory treatment orders. The Act also replaces the nearest relative with a named person who can act as the patient's representative. Community Treatment Orders have to be approved by new Mental Health Tribunals and require the preparation of a care plan by a Mental Health Officer (Atkinson et al., 2005).

Issues of incapacity in Scotland are addressed within the Adults with Incapacity (Scotland) Act 2000, although decision-making capacity is also a factor in the criteria for compulsory detention or treatment in the Mental Health (Care and Treatment) (Scotland) Act, if 'because of the mental disorder the patient's ability to make decisions about the provision of medical treatment is significantly impaired'.

Mental health legislation in Northern Ireland is currently undergoing review and it is expected that the Mental Health (Northern Ireland) Order 1986 and associated legislation will be replaced by a single Act incorporating both mental health and mental incapacity provisions, based on principles of human rights. This unified approach has been broadly welcomed as helping to combat the stigma and discrimination experienced by people with mental health problems (Samuel, 2009; Northern Ireland Executive, 2010).

Implications for Social Work

The complexities of practice when working with people who may be seen as vulnerable or at risk may also raise questions as to which legislation is appropriate in any one situation.

Consider the following from an article in one newspaper:

Mentally ill man dies of hypothermia in housing 'hovel', inquest told

A mentally ill man froze to death in an unheated 'hovel' after social services failed to care for him or clean his home, an inquest heard.
(*Daily Telegraph*, 18 March 2010)

The report describes council officials as being unwilling to force Mayan Coomeraswamy, a 59-year-old man originally from Sri Lanka, to leave his home as this could have been an abuse of his human rights.

Reflection point

Consider the extent to which the powers of the Mental Health Act might be relevant, if at all, in a situation of this kind.
Would any other legislation be relevant in this scenario?
What factors might be involved in weighing up Coomeraswamy's human rights against his need for care?
What is your response to a headline such as this in terms of the language used and underlying attitudes to social care services?

A situation such as this draws our attention to some complex issues involving capacity, mental health and human rights. It also illustrates the very real challenges faced by social workers and other in managing risk, recovery and social justice.

Suffering from a mental disorder does not necessarily mean that someone does not have capacity, and in this case, it may be that Coomeraswamy did not meet the requirements either for compulsory admission to hospital for mental health assessment and treatment, or to be assessed as lacking capacity to make a decision about leaving his home. In terms of human rights he was also entitled to Article 5, the right to liberty, and Article 8, the right to privacy, family life and home.

As well as some suggestion that Section 135 (1) of the Mental Health Act could have been used to remove Coomeraswamy to a place of safety (*Guardian*, 31 March 2010), the use of Section 47 the 1948 National Assistance Act has been referred to as offering a means of removing someone from their home to a hospital or other suitable place on the grounds of insanitary conditions or lack of care, in order to ensure that they receive the attention they require. The period of time concerned is up to three months, with the possibility of further three-month renewals. Earlier debate (Hobson, 1998) has questioned whether public opinion provides sufficient moral justification for the use of this legislation, highlighting the lack of legal safeguards, and both options can also be seen as infringing human rights

It is hard, however, to deny the dilemmas involved in balancing rights against the need for intervention. Perhaps an important element in any situation such as this is the extent to which continuing efforts are made to establish a relationship of trust with the individual concerned, maximizing communication and contact and the potential for a resolution that does not compromise human rights. The question of whether it is preferable to intervene on a statutory basis in order to protect someone's health and wellbeing is ultimately one that is complex.

Concluding Comments

Social work practice is embedded within legislative and policy frameworks, and mental health social work is no exception to this. Users of social work services and carers need social workers to have knowledge about the relevant legislation in order that they can be clear about the services that may be available, the range of possible actions that can be taken within the law and their rights as the recipients of services. Additionally, social workers need to understand and analyse the wider context of social work in order for their practice to be informed by knowledge about trends in health and social care, and for them to make comparisons between different countries and various political and conceptual approaches. An understanding of the historical context of legislation and policy is important, too; this can help to make sense of current developments and to anticipate future changes, as well as the consequences of particular themes or trends. This may also be of importance in understanding the experiences and attitudes of service users and carers that may have been shaped by previous laws and policies no longer operating, but continuing to influence people's thinking. For example, knowledge of an older family member's experience of living in an asylum may affect someone's own willingness to seek help for a mental health difficulty.

In introducing some of the key aspects of the current legislative framework relating to mental health, this chapter has also raised some complex and challenging issues regarding human rights and the difficult decisions that may be involved in balancing the need to promote human rights, dignity and self-determination with the need for the protection and safeguarding of individuals. There are not necessarily any easy or straightforward answers. However, this reinforces the necessity of developing critical and reflective practice that remains focused on human rights and social justice.

Further Reading

Jones, R. (ed.) (2008) *Mental Health Act Manual.* 11th edn. London: Sweet and Maxwell

PART 2

MENTAL HEALTH, INEQUALITIES AND
DIVERSITY

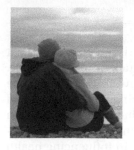

5 Communities and Inequalities

Key points

- The social determinants of health and their relevance for mental health
- Social capital, community and mental health
- The mental health needs of disadvantaged and marginalized groups and communities
- The role of social work in challenging discrimination and promoting social justice
- The social work contribution to mental health promotion with individuals, groups and communities

Introduction

This chapter and the following one form Part 2 of this book in offering an introduction to a range of evidence which is central to a social perspective on mental health, embedded within principles of social justice and human rights. This, it could be argued, is at the heart of the social work contribution to mental health and forms the basis for the chapters that comprise Part 3, where specific aspects of mental health social work practice are explored.

This chapter aims to consider the significance of communities and inequalities for mental health, setting the scene for the specific aspects of diversity that will be considered in Chapter 6.

First some of the evidence concerning the relationship between inequalities, health and mental health will be reviewed, recognizing that this involves the impact of inequalities on mental health and wellbeing, as well as unequal access to services. We will then move on to introduce the concept of social capital and its relevance to mental health.

In relation to social work practice this chapter will address the wider context of mental health, drawing attention to the importance of considering mental health issues outside of 'specialist' mental health social work teams and settings, recognizing the relevance of a community development perspective and the role that social work can play in promoting mental health.

The Social Determinants of Health

When talking about health, whether this be physical or mental, there is often a sense that this is a given and that good health is a matter of chance or good fortune. Similarly, when one is in poor health, it is sometimes considered to be a result of bad luck or just inevitable. Think back to any experience of being unwell, whether it be relatively mild – a recent cold or flu – or something more serious, and you may have made sense of this in terms of an individual explanation such as 'I was a bit run down or stressed.' There may also be a recognition of the part that individual risk factors play in influencing health or ill health, such as smoking or poor diet. Individual behaviours such as these often feature prominently in health promotion campaigns, stressing the need for individual responsibility in promoting and maintaining good health and offering advice on healthy eating and regular exercise.

Thompson (2003) points out that this individualist focus is embedded within traditional medical discourse and that such an emphasis on the individual and individual lifestyle and behaviours effectively conceals underlying issues of social inequality. In relation to mental health, this in turn helps to maintain the predominant influence of the medical model in determining treatment and services, deflecting attention away from the wider environment and the potential for responses at the community or societal level.

There is increasing recognition, however, that social factors are an important influence on health, not simply for individuals but also at the level of groups and communities. Furthermore, this is seen to be crucial in understanding how health issues are understood and addressed and of vital importance for health care professionals and those working in health promotion with individuals and communities. The interrelationship between health inequalities, oppression and discrimination is also a developing theme in social work (Bywaters et al., 2010).

The shift towards the recognition of social factors in health is accompanied by a growing evidence base drawing on both national and international data. A report from the Commission on the Social Determinants of Health (2008) points out that a baby girl born today can expect to live to over 80 in some parts of the world but have a life expectancy of only 45 in others. Such inequalities operate within more affluent countries as well as across the international spectrum. The report states that:

> Where systematic differences in health are judged to be avoidable by reasonable action they are, quite simply, unfair. It is this that we label health inequity. Putting right these inequities – the huge and remediable differences in health between and within countries – is a matter of social justice. Reducing health inequities is, for the Commission on the Social Determinants of Health . . . , an ethical imperative. Social injustice is killing people on a grand scale.   (2008: preamble)

Within the United Kingdom, the findings of the Black Report (Townsend & Davidson, 1988) drew attention to the influence of class differences on health, with higher rates of infant mortality, long-term health conditions and accidents for working-class people. For reasons of political expediency this evidence was downplayed for a number of years. However, similar conclusions highlighting the impact of health inequalities were repeated in subsequent reports (Acheson, 1998; Wanless, 2004). In responding to the Wanless Report, Alan Johnson, then health secretary, made the statement that life expectancy decreases the further east you travel on the London Underground, and that 'For every stop from Westminster to Canning Town, life expectancy goes down one year' (*Guardian*, 9 June 2008).

It would not be cynical to observe that such reports are increasingly charged with recommendations to improve health that are fuelled by financial imperatives to limit and lower levels of public expenditure on health and social care, and have frequently been commissioned by the Treasury. They are also accompanied by messages emphasizing the importance of individuals taking personal responsibility for their own health and the need to combat unhealthy lifestyles. However, as the following statement indicates, there is a continuing theme acknowledging the influence of inequalities on health: 'There are also significant inequalities related to individuals' poor lifestyles and they tend to be related to socio-economic and sometimes ethnic differences' (Wanless, 2004: 4). In referring to ethnic differences this quotation also acknowledges dimensions of inequality other than class and socio-economic factors, and it is important to recognize the socio-economic implications of other aspects of disadvantage and their complex relationship, such as the economic consequences of racism or the poverty experienced by some groups in old age.

While the focus of such reports has tended to be physical rather than mental wellbeing, attention is also being directed towards both the financial and other costs of poor mental health and the interrelationship between mental and physical health, where poor physical health may both contribute to and result from poor mental health. Issues of mental wellbeing are also raised in the Marmot Review of health inequalities in England (Marmot, 2010), which once again highlights the relationship between social and health inequalities. It points to evidence that the **social gradient of health** is particularly pronounced in severe mental health difficulties, showing that for psychotic disorders the prevalence among the population within the lowest quintile of household income is nine times higher than in the highest. The report does acknowledge that this may be affected by downward social drift but suggests that this is unlikely to account for the social gradient. Similarly, scores on the General Health Questionnaire, an assessment that measures psychological wellbeing, also highlight an association between poor mental health and higher levels of deprivation amongst women.

Social gradient of health describes the relationship between health and socio-economic status, where greater affluence is associated with better health.

Reflection point

Identify some of the social factors that may contribute to poor mental health.
  Can you think of any ways in which mental health services might need to change in order to address these issues?

Your responses to the 'Reflection point' will be considered after the following section on access to health care.

Access to Health Care

Social factors can also be seen to play a part in influencing access to health care, having an impact on health and in turn reinforcing the impact of inequality and disadvantage for both individuals and groups. In respect of access to health care it is, however, relevant to note that, unlike other forms of health care, the **inverse care law** does not apply to mental health, where issues of control and coercion in response to concerns about risk can be seen to act as a major influence in some areas of service and care delivery. Portraying mental health care as a continuum, with coercive and controlling influences at one end and supportive and enabling approaches to services at the other, highlights the fact that poorer people and certain Black and minority ethnic groups are over-represented at the former and under-represented at the latter end, as illustrated in Figure 5.1.

Inverse care law
'law' stating that treatment and services are least available for those most in need.

Further discussion regarding some of the evidence regarding the over-representation of certain groups in the figures for compulsory detention under the Mental Health Act will be found in Chapter 6.

Mental Health and Inequality

In responding to the 'Reflection point' in the previous section, it is likely that you will have listed a number of issues that are contained within Figure 5.2, including poverty, poor housing, unemployment,

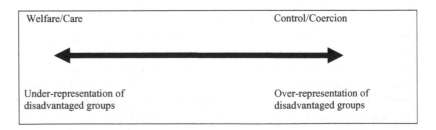

Figure 5.1 The continuum of care and control

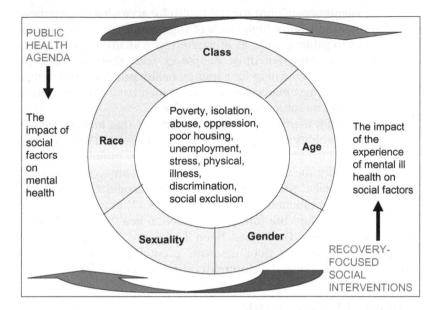

Figure 5.2 The social dynamic of mental health

stress and physical illness, as well as the impact of social exclusion, abuse and discrimination. This figure also portrays the dynamic between those factors that may contribute to mental ill health and the way in which the experience of poor mental health may act to exacerbate or reinforce those very factors themselves, thereby creating a vicious circle from which it may be hard to escape.

Reflection point

Returning to the list of factors that you have already identified as contributing to poor mental health, examine these to consider how poor mental health may in turn affect social and economic status.

One of the factors that may have occurred to you in thinking about this question may be employment status. The evidence suggests that this may not be as straightforward as might be imagined because, whilst unemployment clearly has implications for financial status and hence other issues such as housing and other aspects of quality of life, it is the experience of low pay, insecure work and limited control over work tasks that is most detrimental to mental health (Dooley et al., 2000; Ludermir & Lewis, 2003). The loss of work in terms of being made redundant may also be compounded by other related losses, such as changing routines, reduced social contact, loss of identity, confidence and self-esteem etc. as well as reduced income (Fryer, 1995).

The consequences of poor mental health for accessing employment are also significant, since high levels of stigma and discrimination act as a barrier to gaining work, as illustrated by a snapshot poll undertaken by Mind (2008). For those people in work, there may also be disincentives in seeking help for a mental health problem, including a reluctance to request medical sick notes which record the condition and will need to be submitted to the employer.

More generally, there is considerable evidence that higher levels of psychiatric morbidity and lower longevity are associated with poverty, although as yet the precise causal mechanisms are undefined.

Internationally, the impact of mental health on physical health and vice versa, as well as wider inequalities, is also recognized. The slogan 'no health without mental health' (WHO, 2005: 11) draws attention to this relationship, and the influence of mental health on the Millennium Development Goals has been highlighted, recognizing, for example, the impact of poor maternal mental health on children's physical and emotional development (Miranda & Patel, 2005).

Communities and Health

It will be evident from the discussion so far that, in attempting to understand issues regarding health in general and mental health in particular, we need to consider more than just the individual. In particular we need to broaden our focus to look at groups who may share similar experiences with respect to socio-economic factors, advantage and disadvantage, discrimination and levels of social inclusion or exclusion. In doing so it may be helpful to introduce briefly concepts of social identity and community.

Social identity

This can be understood as a sense of belonging to a social group, involving relationships, interactions and the sharing, or perceived sharing, of certain characteristics, experiences or values. Llewellyn et al. (2008: 47) point out that 'the concept of community may be important in terms of the construction of identity', referring to the concept of *communion* from Lee and Newby (1983), where locality is less important than shared identity and value systems.

Community

The term 'community' has been defined in many different ways by sociologists and others and is often strongly contested. Hoggett (1997: 14) refers to community as a 'fundamentally political concept', stating that the idea of community is 'saturated with power'. This in part refers to the various ways in which the term has been embraced within various political agendas, but also alludes to the tensions inherent in any discussion about community. This is frequently illustrated when questions about where boundary lines are drawn and who belongs are raised. The answers to such questions once again may be seen to reflect a range of issues relating to privilege and power – for example, the 'not in my back yard' response to the setting up of a local service for people with mental health problems or any other excluded group. Such debates benefit from critical deconstruction, challenging commonly held beliefs or assumptions and searching for contradictions, different or missing perspectives and interpretations (Fook, 2002). This might result in new ways of thinking and fresh perspectives, such as the recognition of people already in the 'community' with experience of mental health difficulties, rather than the 'them and us' view that frequently prevails.

The concept of community may also reflect a non-spatial set of relationships. This can be seen in the way in which various groups are developing their use of the internet as a social networking resource, or in the sense of faith groups who may understand themselves as a community that crosses neighbourhood, local or even national boundaries.

Whilst it might appear thus far that a clear definition of community has been avoided, it is hoped that this brief discussion, in the process of drawing attention to the complexities of the term, has also highlighted some common themes relating to a shared sense of identity and belonging with a sense of mutual values and beliefs. As we have already seen in Chapter 2, the need for a sense of belonging and participation is an important factor in mental wellbeing. Conversely, for those people who are not seen as belonging or do not feel included, the lack of 'community' may be associated with social exclusion and stigma.

Social Capital

Recently the term 'social capital' has received considerable attention, both within political discourse and in relation to mental health. Often described as 'the glue that holds society together' (World Bank, 1999), key elements have been identified as a general level of trust, identity, fraternity and networks, contributing to social cohesion. Putnam's (1995) work on social capital has gained particular attention in Britain with a focus on civic renewal and regeneration. Critics, however, have challenged the concept's association with economic interests and productivity and question the notion that this can be progressed without greater attention to more deep-seated inequalities, suggesting that it may obscure cuts in welfare spending and provision (Thompson, 2009).

A particular feature of the theoretical debate concerning social capital is whether or not social capital is a feature of individuals or groups. At an individual level this can be understood in terms of an individual's access to resources such as education or social networks, and as such this can be seen to link to the sociologist Pierre Bourdieu's (1997) view of cultural capital. Tummey and Turner (2008: 31) refer to this as 'knowing one's place' and discuss how this may predict, although not necessarily prescribe, social capital in terms of socio-economic position and social networks etc. In this respect, access to power and to well-paid and high-status employment is likely to perpetuate access to others in a similar position and the benefits that may ensue. Conversely, poor educational qualification, prolonged unemployment and related financial hardship are likely to limit access to influential individuals and networks. This is not to say that access to power and status will remove the risk of mental health difficulties, but such resources may well assist in reducing or ameliorating such risks for some people.

Critics of the individual approach suggest that such a view potentially leaves social capital as a proxy measure for access to social support and networks. An alternative view of social capital is to understand it as embedded within groups and relationships. Such an ecological view is proposed by McKenzie et al. (2002) in a discussion of social capital and mental health.

McKenzie and Harpham (2006) identify three dimensions to social capital:

1. *Structural/cognitive*: 'Structural' describes the number of associations and relationships that exist for any one individual or group, whilst 'cognitive' refers to the values and norms that exist.
2. *Bonding/bridging*: 'Bonding' refers to the inclusive and inward links that exist, for example, within families or very close-knit groups, whilst 'bridging' connects different groups together. It is worth noting that notwithstanding the benefits associated with such close relationships, there are potential disadvantages, as strong inward-looking bonds may lower tolerance towards difference and foster social exclusion for those who do not belong.
3. *Horizontal/vertical*: Horizontal capital links people and groups from the same or similar social strata, whilst vertical social capital connects across different social strata.

Activity

Read the two brief vignettes below and consider the situations of Vanessa and Joseph in relation to the various aspects of social capital that have been discussed.

Vanessa is a well-educated and professionally qualified African Caribbean woman in her thirties. She works for a housing association as a senior manager and lives with her partner, a social worker, and their two children, who attend the local primary school. The death of her sister in a car accident was followed closely by her father receiving a diagnosis of Alzheimer's disease, and Vanessa became very involved in trying to support her mother in caring for her father. Over a period of a couple of months Vanessa became upset and depressed, still grieving for her sister as well as being distressed about her father. Fortunately she was able to renegotiate her working hours to enable her to spend more time with her parents and also accessed a brief period of counselling through an employee assistance programme. Her involvement in local community activities with her children had created a strong social network with other women, and her friends offered her a high level of emotional support as well as practical assistance with child care when she and her partner were not available. Her partner was also able to access information about support for carers and to ensure that the wider family were able to apply for services.

Joseph is a 26-year-old male asylum seeker from Ethiopia. He arrived eighteen months ago and is living in a bedsit in a rundown inner-city area. He has a degree in languages and had wanted to go on to postgraduate study before he left Ethiopia, but since arriving in Britain he has experienced symptoms of post-traumatic stress disorder resulting from the circumstances of his leaving Ethiopia. There are few other Ethiopians in the area that he lives in and his low income means that it is too expensive for him to travel to meet others from the Ethiopian community in a neighbouring town. He has not been able to find work in Britain and spends his time alone, either in his bedsit or walking the streets.

In thinking about these scenarios it may have felt difficult to disentangle ideas of social capital from social networks and social support. Webber suggests that: 'Social capital represents the resources of other people within an individual's social network . . . social support is best perceived from the perspective of the person receiving it' (2005: 102). In this sense, we can see that Joseph's social network is extremely limited and that his access to social capital is therefore similarly limited in comparison with Vanessa's situation. At the same time it is possible to identify the challenges inherent in this conceptual minefield, whilst recognizing the value of attempting to theorize in the area of social relationships, especially in relation to mental wellbeing and social inclusion.

It is acknowledged (Webber, 2005) that, as yet, the measurement of social capital so far is relatively unsophisticated and offers serious methodological challenges to researchers. The concern here, however, has been to consider the relevance of social capital as a concept to assist our understanding of mental health difficulties within both individuals and groups, but also, using that understanding to inform practice, to point to interventions that may promote positive mental health and alleviate difficulties.

Promoting Mental Health

Previous discussion in Chapter 3 has already highlighted the increasing emphasis on promoting mental health embedded within current policy (Department of Health/HM Government, 2009), recognizing the need for a public mental health approach addressing both the overall wellbeing of the population and the prevention and treatment of mental illness. A key message is the need for cross-government working and an integrated approach across health and social care, including statutory and voluntary sector organizations.

The public mental health framework set out in *New Horizons* refers to wellbeing as 'a positive state of mind and body, feeling safe and able to cope with a sense of connection with people, communities and the wider environment' (Department of Health/HM Government, 2009: 18). This definition places mental health firmly within the wide range of life experiences that all social workers encounter in their practice, crossing communities and service areas, regardless of setting or location. However, it may be useful at this point to explore some of these concepts, such as resilience and wellbeing, a little more deeply and to relate them to issues of power and powerlessness, disadvantage and inequality.

Making It Happen, a framework for mental health promotion (Department of Health, 2001a: 30), sets out three levels of intervention; first, strengthening individuals; second, strengthening communities; and third, reducing structural barriers to mental health.

The first level refers explicitly to the building of emotional resilience through 'interventions designed to promote self-esteem, life and coping skills e.g. communicating, negotiating, relationship and parenting skills' (p. 30). At this point it may be helpful to refer to a definition of resilience as a characteristic of individuals, families and communities with 'the ability to withstand or recover quickly from difficulties' and where stress is 'a state of mental, emotional or other strain' (Parrott et al., 2008: 1).

Second, strengthening communities is seen as involving 'increasing social inclusion and participation, improving neighbourhood environments, developing health and social care services which support mental health, anti-bullying strategies at school, workplace health, community safety, childcare and self-help networks' (Department of Health, 2001a: 30). It is important to recognize, however, that, despite many references to mental health at the community level, in reality, as Cattan and Tilford (2006) point out, the majority of this work takes a primarily individual approach. They suggest that this is due, in part at least, to the perceived lack of evidence regarding the effectiveness of interventions targeting the wider determinants of mental health, Indeed this can be seen to mirror a range of public health concerns and priorities where the emphasis is on the need for individuals to take responsibility for their own behaviour and make lifestyle changes in diet and exercise, for example, in order to remain healthy. The difficulties of maintaining a healthy diet or regular exercise for people who are on a low income or who do not have convenient access to safe space or facilities for exercise or to shops with reasonably priced fresh food are rarely acknowledged. Similarly with mental health, the advice offered by various agencies and websites to keep active, eat healthily and talk to others about how you are feeling, whilst helpful at one level, at another perpetuates the idea that mental health is an individual responsibility.

Reflection point

Consider why less attention is paid to interventions to promote mental health at the community level than to those aimed at individuals and families.

Can you identify any interventions or strategies from your own experience that either directly or indirectly contribute to mental health and wellbeing?

In addition to the concerns about the evidence base for community-based interventions, the tension between strategies targeting individual health promotion and wider community-based initiatives reflects wider issues at a governmental level, with the contradiction between the conclusions of the Wanless Report (2004), which pointed to the need to move away from treating illness and to recognize the impact of inequalities, and the messages of *Choosing Health* (Department of Health, 2004a), emphasizing the importance of individual choices in lifestyle and health care (Mackereth & Appleton, 2008).

In reality, programmes intended to improve both physical and mental wellbeing need to be located within a wider understanding of people's lives, embedded within social networks, communities and a range of strategic and structural factors. This recognition that some of the key determinants of health lie outside of the immediate influence of health and social care has led to the description of such factors as 'upstream', with individual lifestyle factors being described as 'downstream', as shown in Figure 5.3.

This means that strategies for mental health promotion need to take into account a wide range of different agencies and organizations, as pointed out in the introduction to *Making It Happen*:

Upstream	General socio-economic, cultural and environmental conditions
Midstream	Living and working conditions
	Social and community influences
Downstream	Individual lifestyle factors
	Age, sex and hereditary factors

Figure 5.3 Upstream, midstream and downstream factors in health
Source: Cameron et al. (2003)

> Many of the factors which influence mental health lie outside health and social care, so mental health promotion is relevant to the implementation of a wide range of policy initiatives, including social inclusion, neighbourhood renewal and health at work. Effective mental health promotion depends on harnessing expertise, resources and partnerships across all sectors and disciplines.
>
> (Department of Health, 2001a: 5)

This emphasis on partnership working is clearly in line with the role of social work, and related issues of multi-agency working will be discussed in Chapter 11.

The third level of mental health promotion interventions includes 'initiatives to reduce discrimination and inequalities and to promote access to education, meaningful employment, housing services and support for those who are vulnerable' (Department of Health, 2001a: 30). In many respects this can be seen to move more into the realm of public policy in areas such as those mentioned – education, housing and employment – clearly going beyond a specifically health agenda. In Britain this can be seen in work that rests outside the Department of Health, often short-lived, such as the Social Exclusion Unit, intended to cut across traditional policy areas. Similarly Health Action Zones were charged with bringing together the various agencies operating in a defined geographical area to work together to improve health outcomes.

Activity

Consider how policy in the arts, housing or transport may have implications for mental health. How, if at all, is this significant for social work practice?

In considering the questions in the activity above, you may, for instance, have thought about the location of housing and how this may help or hinder access to other services. This might mean that a single mother or an asylum seeker finds it difficult to go out and meet other people, thereby increasing their sense of social isolation. Poor-quality housing may be accompanied by costly and inefficient heating systems, increasing the risk of poor physical health and anxiety about money, and generally contributing to a sense of hopelessness and despair. The reduction in the social housing stock also makes it increasingly difficult for people to obtain reasonably priced housing, leaving them no option but to turn to private landlords, in which case there may also be restrictions about offering tenancies to benefit claimants.

You might also have reflected on the extent to which your role as a social worker can take on such issues, your capacity to act as an advocate on such matters or your ability and inclination to become a political activist or campaigner. Working to promote human rights and social justice at the individual level is in itself complex; the prospect of engaging in a level of political activity may be seen as even more challenging.

Community Work

A lengthy discussion on the nature of community work's and social work's involvement in this sphere of activity is beyond the scope of this book. It should nevertheless be noted that social work and community work have often been seen as complementary activities and that historically there has been a strong tradition of working with communities and community development supported by social work principles and practice.

It is relevant, however, to consider the example of Sure Start as a community-based initiative which, whilst created to provide high-quality support for families with young children, can also be seen to have simultaneously been addressing mental health needs, with an emphasis on early parenting, the provision of family support and opportunities for community involvement. It is equally important to recognize the influence of social work and social work values, as the 'Practice example' demonstrates.

Practice example

One Sure Start programme in an area recognized for its high levels of social and economic disadvantage was led by a very experienced social worker with extensive experience of working with children and families. A high level of partnership working involved a Health Trust, Local Authority Early Years and Social Services Departments, and a range of third sector, community-based organizations including a community health organization with a strong tradition of community development work. The programme was also characterized by high levels of participation from local families and residents, including places on the programme management group and involvement in the evaluation of the work, based on a participatory methodology.

Alongside a range of services and interventions designed to support parents and to provide play and child care opportunities for families, there was an identified strand of work that was directly related to supporting mental health in the families involved.

One example included the involvement of the psychologist and health visitor in videoing parents and their young babies to assess levels of bonding and attachment. This also assisted in the early identification of mothers experiencing depression, enabling appropriate support to be offered, including the possibility of referral to a Sure Start counsellor. Mothers were very keen to be involved and enjoyed receiving a copy of the video.

Another example concerns the support offered to families with a child with special needs. The social worker's involvement was highly valued, and both the practical and emotional aspects of her work were acknowledged. This could be seen to have very positive outcomes in terms of the overall wellbeing of the parents, with associated benefits for the children. The mothers themselves commented that they did not know what they would have done without this and suggested that their mental health would clearly have been affected.

This discussion demonstrates how the mental health of families may be promoted by a number of interventions which were ostensibly provided within a 'child care' agenda. It is also important not to underestimate the impact of the style of participation and involvement, which was an essential element of the ethos and practice of the programme. The power relationships engendered by this approach can be seen to set the scene for partnership working and anti-oppressive practice as well as contributing to the building of self-esteem and confidence, in themselves helping to build resilience.

Communities and power

In discussing power, Tew (2005: 71) notes that 'mental distress may often link to experiences of power and powerlessness'. Whilst power is frequently conceptualized as a zero-sum equation, in that there is a finite amount of power to be allocated, like a cake which can be divided into different-sized slices though the cake size remains the same. Instead Tew argues that it can be conceptualized as a social relation between people and viewed as productive in terms of 'power together'. Tew's model of power is set out in Figure 5.4.

Reflection point

Draw on your own experience or practice in communities to identify examples of power from each of the sections of the matrix in Figure 5.4.

What strategies would be required to promote co-operative power and how does this sit alongside other social work roles where protective power may be seen to be necessary?

In respect of mental health, examples of limiting modes of power could include the collusive power demonstrated in campaigns to

	Power over	Power together
Productive modes of power	**Protective power** Deploying power in order to safeguard vulnerable people and their possibilities for advancement	**Co-operative power** Collective action, sharing, mutual support and challenge – through valuing commonality *and* difference
Limiting modes of power	**Oppressive power** Exploiting differences to enhance own position and resources at the expense of others	**Collusive power** Banding together to exclude or suppress 'otherness' whether internal or external

Figure 5.4 Matrix of power relations
Source: Tew (2005: 74)

oppose the location of mental health services in a particular neigh-bourhood, or what has been termed 'not in my backyard' or 'nimby-ism'. This could potentially involve aspects of oppressive power in the use of access to resources such as the media in order to gain further support. This might also move into protective power, as some groups might oppose offering a greater level of independence in terms of housing on the grounds that this would increase risks to vulnerable people in the community. Co-operative power could be seen in the collective efforts of diverse groups to oppose aspects of the mental health legislation proposed by the government before the 2007 Mental Health Act.

Building Networks

Discussion so far in this chapter would suggest that building and strengthening social networks is a key task in promoting mental health. This is further supported by evidence regarding the association between social isolation and depression (Brown et al., 1986; Boreham et al., 2002; Mackereth & Appleton, 2008). Isolation and the absence of support, confiding relationships and 'companionable' activity are not likely to be conducive to positive self-esteem and may create the potential for a vicious circle, whereby low self-esteem makes it more difficult to engage in social relationships, in turn increasing social iso-lation. It is also important to recognize that certain individuals and groups may be more vulnerable to isolation.

Reflection point

Consider which groups and individuals might be more vulnerable to social isolation. How might this impact on their mental health?

In considering the 'Reflection point', it is relevant to remind our-selves of the importance of recognizing the uniqueness of each indi-vidual and the need for a sensitive and collaborative approach in dis-cussing social relationships.

One of the groups that you might have considered is that of people who have experience of mental health problems, who are sometimes neglected when it comes wider issues of mental health promotion. Indeed it may sometimes be difficult to distinguish between interven-tions designed to promote mental health and those intended to address specific difficulties. For the purposes of the discussion in this chapter we will focus on wider interventions with groups or communities (see 'Practice example'), although a 'Practice example' in Chapter 10 will refer to the use of social network maps with individuals.

Practice example

Residents at a mental health hostel were encouraged to join a walking group that was set up by two members of staff. Some of the residents were initially unsure about this activity and lacked confidence in going out or their ability to walk very far. Walks of varying lengths to suit the abilities of the group members were devised, often using public transport to access the countryside. Over time the individuals involved became very committed to the group and increasingly involved in making suggestions for walks and acquiring suitable clothing and footwear to enable them to undertake more challenging routes. A scrapbook was developed with the support of the staff, containing photos and comments about the group's activities which served as a focus for the group outside of the walks and assisted in maintaining social interaction between group members.

There were clearly wider benefits resulting from this initiative in terms of physical health and activity, recognized within the literature as also promoting sleep and increased psychological wellbeing (Callaghan, 2004; Bartholomew et al., 2005). The shared experiences and achievements of the group also contributed to the social relationships of those involved, increasing their sense of self-esteem as valued group members.

Over time the staff hoped to introduce members of the walking group to other community-based activities such as 'Paths to Health' in Scotland, 'Green Gym' or the 'Walking the Way to Health Initiative', described by Morris (2003).

Although at an early stage, findings from research on social capital are also relevant here. However, whilst there is generally a strong sense that belongingness and a sense of connection are an important factor that promotes mental health, the evidence is complex and requires careful consideration. For example, in recognizing the distinction between bonding and bridging forms of capital, Usher suggests that 'The true benefits from social capital stem from the contacts created through bridging across diverse individuals and groups. Within poor minority communities specifically, bridging ties are necessary to break the social economic isolation produced by segregation' (2006: 20). There may also be a personal cost to the individual in the level of obligations required. Whilst this is not to suggest that participation should be discouraged, there is a sense that attention should also be directed towards the development of bridging ties between groups and networks and multiple connections. Evidence from work undertaken with gay men in Australia (McClaren et al., 2008) might support this, finding that the risk of depression was mediated by a sense of belonging to both general and gay communities rather than just to one alone.

There is also a sense that whilst efforts to promote the social inclusion of people with mental health difficulties often challenge their apparent ghettoization within services and activities specific to mental health, a preferable alternative to this dichotomy of mental health or community-based activities might be to acknowledge the benefits of both. For instance, in the 'Practice example' above, members of the walking group within mental health services were encouraged to join similar community-based activities as their confidence increased.

Promoting Resilience

Parrott et al. (2008: 4), in discussing the building of resilience with parents and children, refer to the key components as being a sense of security, a recognition of self-worth and the experience of control over one's immediate environment. In practice these are closely linked to building on strengths and existing coping capacities. The development of effective coping strategies has also been linked to the process of attachment and early relationships, as the earlier example of practice from Sure Start has indicated. Work with children and young people in schools to combat bullying can also be seen to be underpinned by notions of building resilience.

Reflection point

Identify any examples from your own practice or experience where you have contributed to building resilience as part of promoting mental health, or could do so in the future.

What social work skills are required for this work and how do these relate to the key social work roles?

Who else might you work with to develop this work?

Education, Training and Awareness Raising

There may be other opportunities for working with groups and organizations to promote mental health through educational and training initiatives or awareness raising. These might include working in partnership to recognize shared interests and agendas leading to collaborative developments.

'Looked-after' children and young people and care leavers are a group where a high incidence of mental health problems has been identified (Office for National Statistics, 2003). Whilst such issues are often addressed at the level of the individual child or young person, it is useful to consider the options that may be available to promote mental health more widely within this population.

Examples might include providing training and support for foster carers and residential staff working with looked-after children and young people, to enable them to develop a greater understanding of mental health issues and to work with young people in such a way as to promote positive mental health through building self-esteem and efficacy. Lobbying for additional resources to enable looked-after young people to have access to computers or other equipment can be seen as challenging the stigma and disadvantage that many young people experience. Close links with the Children and Adolescent Mental Health Service (CAMHS) might also foster informal relationships with mental health practitioners who might be able to offer advice and information at an early stage when difficulties are identified. Overall, joined-up thinking and planning involving health, education and social care are seen to be crucial (Young Minds, 2006).

Mental health difficulties in older people are often assumed to be related to the onset of dementia. Whilst this is undoubtedly a major concern, there is also justifiable concern regarding levels of depression that remain undetected. Issues of dementia and depression will be explored further in Chapter 8. However, it is relevant here to consider the extent to which ageist attitudes and stereotypes may inhibit accurate assessment and intervention and to consider how these might be challenged, particularly when the dilemma for busy practitioners is often the lack of time for thinking more strategically about community issues.

The particular experiences of Black and minority ethnic communities in relation to mental health, to be considered in Chapter 6, have also elicited interest in developing strategies to work with communities to increase information and raise awareness. Recommendations from the Department of Health's *Inside Outside* document (National Institute for Mental Health in England, 2003) highlighted the need for strategies to work with Black and minority ethnic (BME) communities outside, as well as to address the shortcomings inside mainstream mental health services. References to 'bridging the gap' would seem to echo the earlier discussion regarding social capital, and the role of Community Development Workers was seen to be crucial in working with community groups to tackle health inequalities, through building on existing strengths and capabilities within communities regarding mental health. One such community development team, based within a voluntary sector mental health organization, supported the setting up of self-help groups as well as information giving and mental health awareness raising activities with faith and community groups, working with Irish, Polish, African Caribbean and Asian communities.

For social workers working outside the mental health services, there may be limited opportunities to get involved in such activity. However, an awareness of its value and the ability to make links and connections with other groups are of crucial importance. This may include providing information, signposting or referring individuals to community programmes, recognizing the contribution this can make to promoting mental health.

Mental Health and Inequalities: The Relevance of a Global Perspective

Whilst the main audience for this book is likely to be those working or preparing to work in the UK, it is relevant to turn our attention briefly to the wider context of inequalities and mental health and to recognize the interrelationships and connections between local, national and international issues.

One aspect concerns the ways in which continuing patterns of colonial relationships can be seen in the recruitment of trained staff, including psychiatrists, nurses and social workers, for Western Europe and North America from low-income and middle-income countries. In such countries access to human resources, community services and funding remains limited, and these countries rarely feature in internationally funded mental health research, despite high levels of need (Lancet Global Mental Health Group, 2007; Saxena et al., 2007). Paradoxically there is much that could be learnt by the developed world from developing countries in relation to working with traditional beliefs and practices that could inform thinking about social perspectives and the importance of spirituality and religious beliefs.

Implications for Social Work

Social workers are well placed to make an important contribution to public mental health, not least as a result of their involvement with individuals, families and groups who may already be experiencing disadvantage, and who may be more vulnerable to poor mental wellbeing due to experiences of poverty, physical ill health, abuse and trauma as well as discrimination and oppression.

Opportunities to promote mental health within 'everyday' practice can include working with strengths and building resilience in individuals. Challenging discrimination and stigma and working to promote social inclusion run through all of the various interventions discussed in this chapter, rather like the message in a stick of rock. However, notwithstanding the importance of working with individuals, it is relevant to note the limitations of this strategy inasmuch as such interventions could be seen as reactive in addressing barriers to inclusion as and when they are encountered. A more proactive approach requires making personal links with people in local organizations and keeping in contact in order to maintain relationships that will facilitate access to opportunities in the community. Repper and Perkins (2003: 153) suggest that 'it is preferable to target particular areas rather than trying to change the whole world'; for example, by working with one school to raise awareness or offer support, or building links with employers through one chamber of commerce or one local college.

Activity

Draw a map of your local area. This could be in relation to your place of work or placement or your own home area. Identify any locations which might offer access to community activities, such as the local library, church or sports centre. Be creative in thinking about where opportunities might arise. As part of this exercise, you may wish to take a walk around the local area to see if you can spot other potential possibilities.

Consider how you could contact and build links with some of these resources.

This discussion points to the benefits of social workers having the opportunity to build up their knowledge about the local communities in which they practise. Understanding local issues and being aware of resources and networks is invaluable in developing strategies to promote social inclusion.

Concluding Comments

To return to the theme of social justice, the evidence considered in this chapter offers a brief introduction to the social determinants of health and their significance with regard to mental health and the related issues of inequalities and injustice. These can also be seen to influence access to services, both reflecting and maintaining long-standing issues of disadvantage and discrimination. Such issues are not unfamiliar in any area of social work practice, and the continuing challenge is to identify and counter oppression and discrimination in their many forms. Issues of identity and community also feature strongly in any discussion of mental health and it is important to appreciate the impact of ethnicity, gender, age and sexual orientation, issues that will be explored further in the next chapter.

The introduction of concepts such as social capital into mental health debates is as yet at a relatively early stage and both conceptually and methodologically challenging. Nevertheless, they may contribute to the further development of social work knowledge and practice informed by social perspectives on mental health. There are, however, practical strategies that social workers can adopt to promote mental health within 'everyday' practice. These include taking the time to find out about their own communities and networks, identifying opportunities to build on strengths and creating connections and links between groups and individuals.

Further Reading

Bywaters, P., McLeod, E. & Napier, L. (2010) *Social Work and Global Health Inequalities*. Bristol: Policy Press

McKenzie, K. & Harpham, K. (2006) *Social Capital and Mental Health*. London: Jessica Kingsley

Rogers, A. & Pilgrim, D. (2003) *Mental Health and Inequality*. Basingstoke: Palgrave Macmillan

Tew, J. (ed.) (2005) *Social Perspectives in Mental Health*. London: Jessica Kingsley

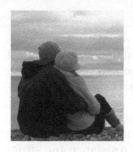

6 Diversity

Key points

- The mental health of Black and minority ethnic groups
- The mental health of lesbian, gay and bisexual communities
- The importance of gender in mental health
- Mental health and the Deaf community
- Developing social work practice that is sensitive to issues of diversity and inequalities

Introduction

In this chapter, the theme of inequalities and the effect on mental health of the social determinants of health introduced in Chapter 5 are considered further in relation to specific areas of discrimination and oppression: the mental health of Black and minority ethnic groups, lesbians, gay men and bisexual people, as well as women's and men's mental health. Reference will also be made to mental health issues as they affect the Deaf community. The literature and research evidence regarding mental health and illness will be examined, including issues regarding access to and the availability of appropriate services.

In turning our attention to specific aspects of oppression and disadvantage it is important to recognize the multifaceted dimensions of identity and community located within the complex lives of individuals. There is no straightforward equation to reveal the sum of various forms of inequality, as in racism + sexism + ageism = X. Instead we are faced with the interwoven texture of separate and related processes that together form the unique experience of any one person. Despite this challenge, a key theme is the impact of oppression on mental health at both institutional and individual levels. It is here that a framework such as that developed by Thompson (2006: 27) may be helpful in differentiating the various levels that will be present in this discussion. In the PCS (personal, cultural and structural) model Thompson identifies the personal and psychological level, the cultural level and the structural or societal level, whilst stressing that these three levels are closely interlinked and constantly interact with one another. Thompson also emphasizes (2003: 178) the need to avoid falling into the trap of focusing on the structural and cultural levels at the expense of the personal, leaving individuals' experience determined entirely by wider influences and lacking any agency of their own. This is particularly helpful in acknowledging that individuals will respond to similar circumstances in many varied ways and that we cannot predict who will be most affected by their experiences of disadvantage or oppression.

The issue of agency raised by Thompson can also be related to Foucault's (1981) thinking about power as being embedded in all social relationships and being manifest in strategies of resistance and struggle against oppression. When considering the experiences of any group that has faced oppression and discrimination, it is essential to remember the strengths and resilience that have been demonstrated as part of the continuing history of striving for recognition and equal rights, and to avoid reinscribing notions of victimhood. Such struggles can also be seen in the experiences of many service users, both individually and collectively, in challenging prejudice and oppressive treatment.

Additionally, we need to question and problematize some of the concepts that may be referred to in this section, as, whilst terms such as 'race', 'lesbian' or 'gay' are in common usage and may be useful in referring to the shared experiences of certain groups of people, they are in themselves open to question. In writing about mental health Fernando (2002: 23) has challenged the notion of 'race' as describing biologically determined categories. Similarly, Hicks contests the use of terms such as 'lesbian' and 'gay' as subscribing to an essentialist view of sexuality. In particular, Hicks (2009) suggests that such terms are part of sexual discourses that shape thinking about sexuality within the privileging of heterosexuality. Gay/straight or Black/White dichotomies can also be seen to obscure other aspects of diversity and maintain 'other'-ness. However, despite these concerns, the identities associated with such language can also be seen to contribute to individuals' claims to a positive self-definition and are central to individual and collective resistance and the development of various liberation movements.

Racism and the Mental Health of Black and Minority Ethnic Communities

Our understanding of the mental health of people from Black and minority ethnic (BME) communities is strongly affected by the discourse of psychiatry and the context within which it developed, when racist attitudes and beliefs were the norm in the predominantly male, White and Western European profession. These included the notion that Black people were inferior and incapable of deeper emotions that might generate depression, as well as the use of psychiatric labelling to justify the medicalization and treatment of behaviour that challenged the status quo.

Additionally, a continuing tension can be found between a form of **cultural relativism** derived from within a particular cultural

Cultural relativism an understanding of a person's behaviour that is embedded within their own culture. This has been seen as leading to the toleration of certain practices which are not accepted in other cultures.

context and a universal approach which, while recognizing some variations in culture, applies a model of psychiatry that fails to understand behaviour fully in its context. Each is problematic in different ways but both function to the disadvantage of the groups concerned.

Looking back in history Fernando refers to examples such as the diagnosis of 'drapetomania', a disease that was seen to be the cause of slaves running away to escape the cruelty and oppression of the slave plantations, and the 1953 work of Carothers, a British psychiatrist who had worked in Kenya, who claimed that depression is rare in Black Africans due to 'the absence of a sense of responsibility' (Fernando, 2002: 104). More recently the diagnosis of 'cannabis psychosis' has been applied predominantly to young Black African Caribbean people in Britain. As Fernando points out, 'It is not necessarily the racial prejudices of individual [research] workers, but the pervasive influence of a racist ideology within which they carry out their work, that is expressed in these theories and ideas' (2002: 101).

The historical influence of racism on psychiatry and the pathologization and over-diagnosis of mental health difficulties in certain BME groups has been viewed as one explanation for the high rates of mental illness found in people from different cultures. Other explanations have been proposed to account for the high rate of mental health difficulties in some BME groups, including the effect of migration. However, in considering the impact of stress on mental health, recent research (Coid et al., 2008) on the incidence of psychosis in first- and second-generation ethnic groups in East London found that the risks were no higher for subsequent generations of immigrants, but that the difference lay between different ethnic groups. The study concluded that it was the presence of protective factors, such as religious and cultural factors as well as family structure, that was effective in buffering stress, again pointing to the significance of social rather than genetic or biological factors, and reinforcing the importance of acknowledging the strengths and resilience of many individuals, families and communities.

The fact remains, however, that people from BME communities experience disproportionately high levels of disadvantage, discrimination and social exclusion when compared to the White population (National Institute for Mental Health in England, 2003) and that these are likely to influence mental health.

Reflection point

Consider the experiences of BME communities in relation to models of mental health based on social construction and social causation.
How does this relate to Thompson's PCS model?

Evidence also indicates that certain BME groups are over-represented within the mental health inpatient population. *Count Me In*, a census of all inpatients in England and Wales undertaken on 31 March 2009 (Care Quality Commission, 2010), found that 22 per cent were from minority ethnic groups. Overall, admission rates were lower amongst White British, Indian and Chinese groups, average for Pakistani and Bangladeshi groups, and higher in Black Caribbean, Black African and other mixed groups. In terms of the route into hospital, the census found that people from Black communities were less likely than those from White groups to be referred to hospital by their GP or by a Community Mental Health Team, but more likely to enter hospital from the criminal justice system. Additionally, people from Black and mixed White–Black groups were seen to be three times more likely than average to be detained under the Mental Health Act, with rates for women from Black Caribbean, Black Africa and Other Black groups between 56 per cent and 62 per cent higher than average.

It is also relevant here to refer to the experiences of the Irish communities in Britain, which have a not dissimilar profile to Black African and African Caribbean groups in relation to their over-representation in certain aspects of service provision, but whose experience is often invisible (Bracken et al., 1998). The 2009 *Count Me In* census (Care Quality Commission, 2010) found that White Irish people were more likely to be on medium or high secure wards than their non-Irish White counterparts.

Work by Audini and Lelliott (2002) found that the rate of civil detentions under the Mental Health Act was six times higher for Black people than White people, with rates of 450 per 100,000 and 68 per 100,000 respectively, and eight times higher for Black men than White men. The rate for Asian people was also higher than that for White people, at 112 per 100,000. This evidence supports the exception to the inverse care law that was referred to in Chapter 5, pointing to the over-representation of certain BME groups in aspects of services that are controlling and coercive, and their under-representation in less restrictive routes to care and treatment.

Reflection point

What explanations might there be for the over-representation of BME people within inpatient mental health services?

In thinking about the 'Reflection point' you may have considered some of the following:

- higher prevalence of severe mental illness within BME groups;
- delays or difficulties in accessing services at an early stage;
- poor compliance with medication;

- greater contact with the police;
- discriminatory responses from services and workers.

Some of these have been seen as contributing to 'circles of fear', a phrase used in the title of a report from the Sainsbury Centre for Mental Health (2002). This describes a pattern of services becoming involved only at the point of crisis and when issues of risk and control become a greater focus of attention, in turn increasing the fear of mental health services. This is seen to result, at least in part, from experiences of oppressive, restrictive and culturally insensitive mental health care that acts as a deterrent to people accessing support for mental health difficulties at an early stage.

One incident that particularly drew attention to the experience of mental health treatment received by non-White groups was the death of David Bennett, an African Caribbean patient in a secure unit, who died in 1998 after being restrained by six nurses. The independent inquiry following David Bennett's death concluded with a number of recommendations including the need for the mental health workforce to reflect diverse communities, training to increase cultural awareness and sensitivity, strategies for tackling racism, the integration of ethnic origin and cultural needs into the Care Programme Approach, and further guidance and training on restraint. The report also recommended the need for 'Ministerial acknowledgment of institutional racism in the mental health services and a commitment to eliminate it' (Blofeld et al., 2003: 67).

The publication of the *Inside Outside* report (National Institute for Mental Health in England, 2003) initiated a process of reform both to improve the capability of the mental health workforce to offer culturally sensitive services, and to increase the capacity of communities for dealing with mental ill health with greater information and more effective engagement. The acknowledged deficit in the availability of culturally and linguistically sensitive services raises issues of citizenship and entitlement which continue to require serious attention, and which for Sewell raises the concern that, without action being taken to address inequalities within mental health services, '*the default position is likely to be continued inequality*' (Sewell, 2009: 39).

Reflection point

Consider what action could be taken by mental health teams and practitioners to address issues of inequality affecting people from BME groups.

One example of work to improve access to mental health services for one minority ethnic group can be found in the 'Practice example' below.

Practice example

The Enhanced Pathways in Care Project in Sheffield is part of the national Delivering Race Equality programme, working with the Pakistani community to build links between the community and statutory mental health services.

The project is based on an already established Pakistani Muslim Centre which lies at the heart of the community, providing a venue for a wide range of social and cultural activities.

Contact was made with the imams and other community leaders to discuss how the centre could be involved in providing mental health services. It now offers a range of activities to support people experiencing mental health difficulties, including cookery and exercise classes. The centre also works with the home treatment service as well as raising mental health awareness (Community Care, 2008).

The objective of increasing trust and engagement is at the heart of efforts such as this to improve the experiences of BME individuals and groups in terms of overall mental health and wellbeing, access to services and the availability of effective care and treatment within a recovery-focused paradigm.

In considering the need for mental health services that are culturally sensitive to the needs of diverse groups, Fernando highlights the risks inherent in focusing on the oppressed rather than the oppression as the problem, thereby perpetuating a deficit model which 'has the effect of pathologising and stigmatising the oppressed' (2002: 107). In a similar vein, Sachidaran (Bhui & Sachidaran, 2003: 11) warns against prioritizing difference over inequality, emphasizing the continuing challenge of addressing institutionalized racism, rather than focusing on 'special needs' within what he describes as the 'colonial discourse of transcultural psychiatry'.

Within such an approach, the potential strengths of Black individuals and their families, sometimes forged through the experience of oppression, remain invisible, despite the various forms of collective political activism and social movements which have served to challenge and continue to challenge all forms of oppression and discrimination. Bowl (2007) also stresses the need for a commitment to change, paying greater attention to the experiences of Black service users who continue to feel that their voices are not heard.

Lesbian and Gay Mental Health

When considering issues of sexuality and the mental health of lesbians and gay men, there are some parallels with the way in which psychiatry has responded to issues of 'race' and culture. A key aspect of this concerns the way in which lesbians and gay men have been pathologized within a model of psychiatry that is underpinned by the privileging of heterosexuality.

Same-sex behaviour and relationships have endured religious preju-dice, moral censure and legal proscription, being viewed as sinful, immoral and illegal at various points through history. Overall, however, much of the attention has focused on male homosexuality, with women's same-sex relationships remaining invisible. Throughout Europe the death penalty was invoked for sodomy, with legislation in England being introduced in 1533. This penalty was lifted only in 1861, although this did not lead to acceptance but rather to continuing le-gislative censure, with 'the commission by any male person of any act of gross indecency with another male person' being made illegal by the Criminal Amendment Act of 1885. This legislative censure was further supported by increasing medicalization of homosexuality, as psychia-try and psychology continued to strive to develop their scientific basis. The development of 'sexology' pronounced homosexuality to be a bio-logical condition requiring treatment, including castration, hormone treatment and aversion therapy, with such attempts at 'cure' continu-ing well into the twentieth century (King & Bartlett, 1999).

Reflecting on the period of recent history in Britain, the picture has been one of pathologization or invisibility. It is only in the last century that terms such as 'lesbian' and 'gay' have come into common usage to describe sexual orientation, although, as already pointed out in this chapter, it is also relevant to consider the part that language and cat-egorization play in maintaining **heteronormativity** and the patterns and practices of power and privilege associated with fixed categories such as lesbian or gay.

Heteronormativity ways of thinking about sexuality that privilege heterosexuality.

Despite the legalization of homosexuality in 1967, theoretical models in psychiatry and psychology continued to emphasize abnormality, justifying the continuation of oppressive practices and so-called treat-ments. After a process of lobbying and campaigning, homosexuality was removed from the Diagnostic and Statistical Manual (DSM) in the USA in 1973 and from the International Classification of Diseases (ICD) in 1992, but the diagnosis remained on the British database of mental illnesses until 1994. Carr, writing about her treatment from a psychotherapist, states that:

> By the end of the first consultation the therapist had discovered my sexual orientation which provided him the disease to cure and because I was not at all that happy about my sexuality at that stage I complied with him. Thus our therapeutic project became my 'hetero-sexualisation', the idea being that if I became heterosexual then I would be cured of my mental distress. So my homosexuality was my illness.   (Carr, 2005: 169).

It is important not to place the entire responsibility for such practices on psychiatry and psychology, however, as they need to be understood as both reflecting and further legitimizing homophobic and heterosex-ist attitudes and behaviour within wider society. Returning to Foucault

(1965), we can see once more the role that the 'psy complex' plays in the regulation of society.

Despite the decriminalization of male homosexuality in 1967 (Sexual Offences Act), the legalization of civil partnerships (Civil Partnership Act 2004) and the legal protection offered by new legislation such as the Equality Act (Sexual Orientation) Regulations 2007, as well as the presence of openly gay and lesbian politicians and sports and media personalities in public life, there is continuing evidence of heterosexism and homophobia, including physical violence.

Homophobia and bullying in schools remain a serious concern, sometimes with far-reaching and damaging consequences for young people, with high rates of suicide and self-harm being found particularly among young gay people (Rivers, 2001, 2004). With respect to educational achievement and future qualifications and employment, bullying and violence were found to increase levels of absenteeism and lead to a greater chance that young lesbians and gay men would leave school at age 16 even after achieving the equivalent of six GSCEs at grade C. This may lead to longer-term disadvantage and have the potential for further contributing to issues of stress and poor mental health (Equalities Review, 2006). There is also evidence of bullying, fear of bullying and poor expectations of health care amongst adults (Hunt & Dick, 2008).

The concept of internalized homophobia (Bremner & Hillin, 1994) has been used to describe the way in which, in the absence of positive images, role models and attitudes, gay men and lesbians develop internalized negative messages about themselves, with the potential to lead to low self-esteem, self-abuse, depression and anxiety. Work undertaken by King and McKeown (2003) found that gay men and lesbians reported more psychological distress than heterosexual men and women, with higher levels of substance and alcohol abuse. Subsequent research (King et al., 2007) suggests that the risks of alcohol and other substance dependence are one and a half times greater than in the heterosexual population, with lesbian and bisexual individuals particularly at risk.

A systematic review commissioned by the National Institute for Mental Health in England pointed to the increased risk of suicide attempts amongst lesbian, gay and bisexual people, with gay and bisexual men being found to be four times as likely to attempt suicide as heterosexual men (King et al., 2007). Following the publication of this review, lesbian, gay and bisexual people have now been included as a specific group within the National Suicide Prevention Strategy for England (National Mental Health Development Unit, 2009).

Although there is little information regarding variability within the lesbian, gay and bisexual population, work by Meyer et al. (2008) in New York found a higher rate of attempted suicide amongst Black and Latino than amongst White lesbians, gay men and bisexuals. Overall this study also found lower rates of stress and mood-related difficulties

amongst younger people, pointing to a suggestion that increasing lib-
eralization may lead to a decline in such problems.

In terms of access to services, gay men and lesbians are more
likely than heterosexuals to have consulted mental health professionals in the past, and among those who had consulted mental health
professionals, up to a third of gay, a quarter of bisexual men and over
40 per cent of lesbians recounted a negative or mixed response from
mental health professionals when open about their sexuality (King &
McKeown, 2003). These findings reflect earlier work (McFarlane, 1998)
showing that while many lesbians and gay men reported avoiding
services or not feeling safe enough to be 'out' when consulting mental
health professionals, others experienced negative responses including
physical or verbal abuse, voyeurism, stereotyping or the trivializing of
relationships. The need to build trust in services is a recurrent theme
running through this and other research, as is the challenge of asking
about sexual orientation when service users are first referred.

Reflection point

What is your view about asking service users about their sexual orientation?
  Are there times when this might be more or less helpful?
  What skills and knowledge do you consider are needed to respond appropriately to lesbians,
gay men and bisexual people experiencing mental health difficulties?

In concluding this section on the mental health of lesbians, bisexuals and gay men it is relevant to revisit the notion of community. There
can often be a tendency to highlight the difficulties and stresses associated with being lesbian, gay or bisexual, and whilst these are undoubtedly real, it is equally necessary to recognize the strengths and resources
that exist within these communities and the various ways in which
these help to build resilience and positive mental health. Referring
back to the earlier discussion of social capital, it is also interesting to
note that one small-scale Australian study (McLaren et al., 2008) found
that, for gay men, a sense of belonging to both gay and general communities mediated the risk of depression. Life for the majority of lesbians and gay men in Britain revolves around the network of friends
and family, of choice and/or birth, and purposeful activities that contribute to mental health and wellbeing, regardless of sexuality.

Gender and Mental Health

Women's mental health has been the focus of critical inquiry for a
number of years. By comparison the field of men's mental health is less
well developed and is only now receiving attention. This distinction
between men's and women's mental health itself merits further

attention, and will be considered before moving on to discuss issues which relate specifically to either men or women.

First, however, we shall consider some of the facts and figures that denote women's and men's mental health in terms of incidence of mental health difficulties and also admissions to hospital under the mental health legislation. A report on psychiatric morbidity among adults living in private households (McManus et al., 2009), based on a survey of individuals aged 16–74 years in England, Wales and Scotland, found that nearly a fifth of women were seen to have a common mental disorder, with a rate of 19.7 per cent, peaking between the ages of 45 and 64, whereas the rate for men was 12.5 per cent. This applied across all diagnostic categories including depression and anxiety, with the exception of panic disorder and obsessive-compulsive disorder. Rates were also found to be higher for White, Black and South Asian women than for White, Black and South Asian men. For psychotic disorders in the preceding twelve months, the overall prevalence was 0.3 per cent for men and 0.5 per cent for women. Additionally, 9.2 per cent of women and 3.5 per cent of men screened positive for eating disorders.

Hospital admission rates also reflect differential rates of access to services, with fewer inpatient beds being occupied by women than by men, although women from Black groups were twice as likely as White women to be admitted, with higher rates for White Irish women than White British women. The rates for White British, Indian and Pakistani groups, however, were lower than average. These differences are also reflected in detentions under the Mental Health Act, where, of those inpatients surveyed overall, 46 per cent of men and 29 per cent of women had been compulsorily admitted, with rates of 56–62 per cent for women from Black Caribbean, Black African and other Black groups (Commission for Healthcare Audit and Inspection, 2005).

The *Mental Health Bulletin* (NHS Information Centre, 2008a) also reported higher numbers of men (54,900) than women (51,600) as hospital inpatients in the year 2006–7, with older women more heavily represented. At the same time more women (512,000) than men (413,500) were found to be using outpatient and community mental health services. Men were also more likely than women to be detained under the Mental Health Act and formed a significantly higher proportion of those detained via the criminal justice system.

Attempting to make sense of these figures, however, raises questions about how mental health is understood and the extent to which notions of gender are embedded within notions of mental health and illness, with Prior commenting that 'the social construction of mental disorder, as reflected in measures of psychiatric morbidity and diagnostic categories, tended . . . to make women highly visible and men almost invisible' (1999: 81). Prior argues that the apparent over-representation of women in these figures begins to disappear if alcohol and substance use are included. This is illustrated by findings from the UK national survey already referred to that indicate the higher prevalence of hazardous drinking among men (33.2 per cent) than among women (15.7 per cent), and that overall 12 per cent of men and 6.7 per cent of women reported using illegal drugs in the preceding year. Prior's analysis included data from the USA, where greater attention to psychosomatic disorders and substance abuse led to the finding that men had a higher lifetime prevalence than women – 36 per cent and 30 per cent respectively – and the same annual prevalence rate, leading Prior to the conclusion that such research evidence supports the feminist allegation of institutionalized sexism in social definitions of mental disorders.

An additional point to consider is the changing landscape of mental health services. In particular the redirection of attention towards community-based services and a reduction in the number of inpatient beds, alongside increasing concerns with risk, have, in effect, increased the risk of hospitalization for men, who may be perceived to be more potentially dangerous. At the same time there is a risk that women's access to services may be reduced and their needs neglected (Payne, 1999).

Women and mental health

Williams (2005) summarizes the factors influencing women's mental health as follows:

- access to resources that promote mental health;
- greater exposure to mental health risks;
- processes that maintain the status quo.

The discussion that follows will begin by considering the processes that maintain the status quo and posing the questions put forward by Williams in relation to both women and men, asking what is it to be a 'good' man or woman and how notions of masculinity and femininity influence mental health.

Referring back to Thompson's PCS model, we can identify the various ways in which these messages form part of a discourse of gender which shapes our thinking about ourselves as gendered beings and our consequent thoughts and behaviours. At the structural level we become aware of the various power differences and inequalities that exist between women and men, whilst at the cultural level a complex set of norms and expectations are seen to influence what is understood to be 'normal'. These are also present in terms of thoughts, feelings and attitudes at the personal or psychological level.

Reflection point

Consider from your own experience the messages you have received regarding what it is to be a 'good' man or woman. Reflect on how these may have influenced your own and others' mental health.

One example that might arise from the 'Reflection point' is the conventional views about emotionality for women and men. Some of you may have considered the view that men are not expected to show their vulnerability and emotions related to sadness or distress, although expressions of joy and achievement in sport, for example, or of anger, may be more acceptable in that they do not challenge the commonly held views about being a proper man. Conversely for women, tears and sadness may be more acceptable whilst the outward demonstration of anger may be less so. Such behaviours and associated expectations may of course vary across cultures. However, the point remains that any such expectations, linked to societally and culturally expected notions of behaviour, have the potential for creating concern when challenged. Such concern may be manifest at a number of levels, within the family or community, or within wider institutions such as schools, or within health care and psychiatry. In this sense, gender and the implications for mental health are socially constructed.

Whilst it is possible to imagine a world where such differences in gender expectations do not result in differential treatment and behaviours towards women and men, a review of what it is to be a healthy person would suggest that the characteristics associated with being masculine or feminine are not equally valued. A study by Broverman et al. (1970) found that whilst the characteristics associated with masculinity were inherently viewed as positive and healthy, those associated with women were seen as unhealthy, leading Chesler to conclude that 'Women, by definition, are viewed as psychiatrically impaired – whether they accept or reject the female role – simply because they are women' (Chesler, 1989: 115). In support of this are many examples of the ways in which women who challenged the conventional role expected of them were treated, including the incarceration in asylums of women who had illegitimate children (Showalter, 1987; Appignanesi, 2008). Such practices both arose from and maintained ideas regarding the feminization of mental illness related to cultural and historical notions of madness and hysteria. In the process, the space for men to demonstrate their vulnerability in terms of psychological distress was confined within narrow boundaries, and primarily legitimized in relation to men experiencing trauma as a result of war.

Williams's (2005) second point concerns women's greater exposure to mental health risks, a factor acknowledged by the Department of Health's (2002b) document on mainstreaming women's mental health, which also highlighted the impact of such risks on women's mental wellbeing. Offering a strategic approach to mental health care for women, the report addressed links between the social and economic context of women's lives, mental health and needs for support or treatment, and also identified groups of women who may be particularly vulnerable, including older women, women in prison, lesbian and transsexual women, women from BME communities, sex workers, mothers and carers, and those with learning difficulties or using alcohol or other substances.

Women's mental health is also more likely to be affected by the experience of violence and abuse, with a recognized association between domestic violence, depression, post-traumatic stress and self-harm (WHO, 2001; Humphreys & Thiara, 2003). It is estimated that at least half of the women using mental health services in the UK and the USA have experienced sexual or physical abuse as children and/or as adults (Itzen, 2006).

Additionally, it is important to recognize that for many women work is devalued and unpaid, with many undertaking unpaid caring responsibilities within the family. Women frequently bear the majority of the burden of child care responsibilities and housework whilst having less control over finances and other household matters than their male partners. This is linked to evidence concerning the relationship between poverty and mental health (Sheppard, 2002).

In looking at exposure to mental health risks, it will be clear that the discussion has again moved from a model based on social construction to one based on social causation, suggesting that neither model is sufficient on its own to make sense of gender and mental health and that, as already stated, in Ussher's words:

> There can be no simple answer to the question of whether women's madness is a misogynistic construct, or a mental illness. It is both. It is neither. It cannot be encapsulated within one explanation, one interpretation. As women, we are regulated through the discourse of madness. But the woman herself is real, as is her pain – we must not deny that. So we must listen to women.   (1991: 306)

Returning to Williams's first point, namely access to resources that promote mental health, she points to stark differences in women's access to money and the greater likelihood that women, especially lone parents and older women, will live in poverty. Linked to this are issues of access to and opportunities for employment, recognizing that women are more likely to be found in low-status and low-paid occupational areas with less access to training. Underlying these factors is the continuing impact of the various ways in which women are treated as being of less value than men, and the accompanying messages that focus on women's sexual and reproductive capacities, a point recognized internationally by the World Health Organization (WHO, 2001), commenting on women's lesser access to social and political power, health, education and employment.

These themes can also be identified in relation to women's experiences of mental health services, where efforts to challenge the provision of mixed-sex wards are still continuing as part of a campaign to ensure women's safety in hospital. As an alternative, women state that they need greater access to talking treatments and alternatives to hospital admission, greater sensitivity to the impact of violence and abuse, and need to feel valued and respected for their strengths and resources: 'the efficacy of mental health services rests on their capacity to provide respectful and safe relationships within which women can tell their own stories of disempowerment and survival' (Williams, 2005: 164).

Men's mental health

It is interesting to consider the reasons for a new and growing interest in men's mental health, which has previously received little attention. Concern in Britain in response to an increasing suicide rate, especially amongst young men, issues of risk and danger and the high rate of mental health issues to be found in the offender population can be seen as contributory factors, although other influences may be relevant.

In relation to exposure to mental health risks for men, one area concerns the risk of unemployment, with evidence suggesting that approximately one in seven men who become unemployed will develop a depressive illness in the following six months. Additionally, unemployment was found to be associated with a doubling of the suicide rate, and lack of job security was found to be a risk factor (Lewis & Sloggett, 1998).

Overall suicide rates for men have also caused concern, with figures for 2008 showing 17.7 per 100,000, compared to a rate of 5.4 per 100,000 for women. This forms part of an overall downward trend in the number of male suicides, which peaked at 21.1 per 100,000 in 1992 and 1998 (Office for National Statistics, 2010). Further analysis also reveals that married men are less likely to commit suicide, and half of the increase in young male suicide may be due to the fact that fewer young men are married. Men who are divorced, separated, widowed, unemployed or shy are seen to be most at risk.

In considering men's mental health, *Men Behaving Sadly*, a report from the Royal College of Psychiatrists (1998), highlighted concerns regarding issues of risk and dangerousness and men's emotional health, in terms of their capacity and opportunity for the expression of feelings. The report also suggested that, contrary to the evidence referred to above, depression rates for men are equal to those of women but that women are diagnosed and treated twice as often. This suggests that not only are women subject to institutionalized sexism in the process of diagnosis and treatment in that they are over-represented, but men are also disadvantaged through being excluded or overlooked in access to treatment and services. This can also be seen in the Goldberg and Huxley (1992) diagram introduced in Chapter 2 (Figure 2.1), showing access to mental health services from the community to specialist services. Within this, women were seen to be more likely than men to be recognized as having mental health difficulties at the primary care stage, but less likely than men with comparable difficulties to be referred on to specialist mental health services.

A report published in 2010 (Wilkins, 2010) draws together a range of evidence and concerns regarding men's mental health, highlighting the potential under-diagnosis of depression, continuing high rates of suicide and the needs of particularly vulnerable groups including prisoners and ex-servicemen. A key message from this report is that being male increases your chances of drug and alcohol dependency, school failure and exclusion, suicide and involvement in crime. It also points to the high rates of mental disorder amongst men in prison and the fact that men are the majority of those detained in secure mental institutions.

Notwithstanding the legitimate concerns regarding men's mental health and the importance of considering how services can best respond, Featherstone et al. (2007) offer a note of caution in responding to universalist notions of male characteristics, and instead emphasize socially constructed aspects of gender identity and practice, challenging any emerging discourse of victimhood. They suggest that whilst 'limited emotional repertoires' in some men may limit or cause tension in relationships, emotional distance can also be seen as facilitating social dominance and male achievement.

The Deaf Community

One group whose mental health needs are rarely highlighted is that of Deaf and hard-of-hearing people, where it is estimated that 40 per cent of people experience mental health difficulties at some point in their lives, being at higher risk for depression and anxiety than the hearing population (Kram & Loeb, 2007; Turner et al., 2007). There is also some evidence to suggest that the rates of paranoia and paranoid psychosis are higher in those who acquire deafness in middle age (SIGN/Mental Health Foundation, n.d.).

In terms of disadvantage, Deaf children are more likely to experience emotional, physical or sexual abuse than hearing children and may also encounter barriers in accessing education, training and employment as adults, with consequences for material and emotional wellbeing and social inclusion (ADSS, 2002; Bradshaw, 2002). The mental health risks for the 90 per cent of Deaf children of hearing parents are greater than for those children born to Deaf parents, who have been found to have higher self-esteem (National Institute for Mental Health in England, 2005b).

There are also recognized barriers to services, particularly in terms of Deaf awareness and the lack of British Sign Language (BSL) interpreters (National Institute for Mental Health in England, 2005b). As we have already seen with some other groups, as well as having a high level of unmet need, Deaf people are over-represented in secure facilities, and it is acknowledged that Deaf offenders with mental health difficulties may initially be let off or cautioned, especially in the absence of BSL interpreters, but may then go on to commit more serious offences leading to imprisonment or secure mental health facilities (Kitson & Thacker, 2000). Recommendations for improvements include greater access to specialized staff and services, increasing the numbers of Deaf people employed in mental health services, and generally extending the capacity of staff in terms of awareness and BSL communication and interpretation.

For social workers, working with Deaf people also requires an understanding of the unique experiences and rich traditions and resources of the Deaf community, whose language and culture engender a sense of pride in its members.

Implications for Social Work

In considering the implications of the various aspects of inequality and diversity presented in this chapter, it is important to hold simultaneously in mind both the wider picture of the various ways in which certain groups have been treated historically and continuing experiences of oppression and discrimination, whilst also recognizing the uniqueness of any one individual and their specific experiences and circumstances. The following statement by Cosis Brown in relation to the needs of lesbians and gay men can be seen as having wider relevance for any particular group that may have experienced oppression, and highlights the central importance of building relationships at the heart of social work practice:

> What lesbians and gay men want . . . is that they are treated the same as all receivers of . . . services, at the same time as some of the very real differences being acknowledged . . . to be seen as a unique individual within her/his own social and political current and historical context.
>
> . . . To work effectively . . . requires this radical approach as it requires the ability to work with contradictions, to use the law as leverage to meet people's needs, to apply knowledge effectively and to utilise competently communication skills in relationship-based work.
>
> (Cosis Brown, 2008: 273)

For social workers, developing an understanding of an individual's history and experience is an intrinsic and essential element in building relationships that can transcend unidimensional notions of identity based solely on ethnicity, gender, sexuality, age, faith or religion.

Concluding Comments

This chapter has examined specific aspects of diversity and inequality in relation to the mental health of people from Black and minority ethnic groups, lesbians and gay men, women and men and also the

Deaf community. Issues of social construction and social causation, as introduced in Chapter 2, have been seen to be relevant to the experiences of groups that continue to face oppression and discrimination in their everyday lives, and to the detrimental consequences of this for their mental health and access to services.

For social workers, acknowledging the complexity and the multidimensional nature of identity in relation to gender, ethnicity and sexuality is essential. This requires holding in mind an understanding of the broader social context that impacts on people's lives with regard to racism, homophobia etc., whilst also paying attention to the uniqueness of any one person's experience. Listening to those experiences and individual stories contributes to the development of relationships that, in turn, are central to practice that is focused on promoting well-being and recovery.

Further Reading

Fernando, S. (2002) *Mental Health, Race and Culture*. 2nd edn. Basingstoke: Palgrave Macmillan

Fish, J. (2006) *Heterosexism in Health and Social Care*. Basingstoke: Palgrave Macmillan

Sewell, H. (2009) *Working with Ethnicity, Race and Culture in Mental Health*. London: Jessica Kingsley

Wilkins, D. (2010) *Untold Problems*. London: National Mental Health Development Unit/Men's Health Forum

PART 3

SOCIAL WORK PRACTICE AND
MENTAL HEALTH

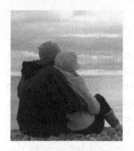

7 The Mental Health of Children, Young People and Families

Key points

- Promoting the development of mental health in families with young children
- The mental health of parents
- Addressing the mental health of young people
- Children and young people as carers

Introduction

This chapter will consider how social workers can identify and begin to respond to a range of mental health issues that may be encountered in any social work setting when working with children, young people and families. A theme in this and the following chapter will be the relevance of a life course perspective that recognizes how the events and experiences of one life stage may influence and affect later experiences. In particular, the potential lasting effects of socio-economic disadvantage will be acknowledged as having a cumulative impact, 'not an event that strikes at a single point' (Graham & Power, 2004: 1). At the same time it is important to avoid a deterministic stance towards those experiencing adverse circumstances, offering no hope for positive change in the future. The positioning of people as passive victims, for example as a consequence of poverty or abuse, whilst on the one hand recognizing the effects of events beyond their control, needs to be replaced by an approach that promotes a sense of efficacy and resilience. In relation to young people, Cattan and Tilford (2006: 105) define resilience as 'a holistic process involving positive mental health of young people within the context of their lives, shaped by their varying skills and the environment, contributing to a hopeful future in the face of adversity'.

For social workers it is especially important that a clear rationale is available to support the longer-term benefits of particular interventions as a counter to the pressure to meet immediate targets and outcomes. Friedl (2009: 41) suggests that respect and justice are the public mental health equivalents of sewers and clean water for physical wellbeing. These principles surely suggest that social workers are placed in a key position to make a significant contribution to promoting mental health wherever they are working.

When reading this chapter there will also be reminders to think about the social construction of the various terms used, such as 'childhood' and 'family'. For example, the use of the term 'family' needs to be understood in relation to a specific physical and temporal location, rather than assumed to be a constant and never-changing concept. Similarly, whilst 'childhood' may be associated with notions of innocence and lack of responsibility, there are many examples across the world and over time which locate children as important contributors to family income through child labour, or in performing key tasks to support the family such as caring for livestock or fetching water. Whilst the readers of this text may be largely UK-based, it is worth acknowledging that the cosmopolitan and international nature of the population in Britain includes many communities with recent and diverse experiences of life elsewhere. These also need to be understood in the wider picture of inequalities influenced by global policies across a number of areas, including foreign policy, health, trade and immigration, acknowledging for example the experiences of street children or those who are trafficked or involved in prostitution (Baldwin, 2009).

The chapter will begin by considering a mental health perspective on social work with children and families, recognizing the sometimes conflicting demands that may arise between addressing the needs of parents and those of children. For example, this might be found where a single mother is finding it difficult to cope with her two young children and there are concerns for their wellbeing. A response which focuses solely on the needs of the children may neglect the mother's own mental health needs, and vice versa. In such situations it is essential to bear in mind, at all times, the principles that the child's needs are paramount. However, a thoughtful and creative approach may enable the needs of all family members to be addressed. We shall then turn to look at the mental health of young people in adolescence and the transition to adulthood. In each section some of the common challenges that may characterize this group as well as key mental health issues that may arise in this area of work will be addressed. A brief introduction to a range of intervention strategies will also be outlined, as well as linking with Chapter 5 in considering ways to promote mental health and to build resilience as an integral element of social work practice. When reading this chapter it will also be important to make your own connections across the various sections, responding to prompts in the text that will challenge the compartmentalization of issues.

Mental Health Difficulties in Childhood

Figures indicate that 10 per cent of 5–15-year-olds in Britain have a recognizable mental health disorder, suggesting that over a million children and young people would benefit from specialist mental health services. Of these, up to 45,000 children and young people are seen to have a severe mental health disorder. Such problems may be associated with educational difficulties, family disruption, disability, offending and anti-social behaviour, with longer-term consequences for future adult life. Overall it is estimated that approximately 40 per cent of these children are not currently receiving any specialized services (Department of Health, 2004c; Green et al., 2005).

Mental health difficulties in children are grouped into three main areas:

- *conduct disorders*, characterized by behaviour that is awkward and troublesome, aggressive or anti-social;
- *hyperactivity*, including inattention and overactivity;
- *emotional disorders*, including anxiety, depression and obsessions.

A survey of over 10,000 children and young people in Britain in 2004 (Green et al., 2005) found that 5 per cent of those surveyed had a conduct disorder, 4 per cent were assessed as having emotional disorders and 1 per cent had hyperactive disorders. Certain groups were also found to be more vulnerable, including 'looked-after' children, who are five times more likely to experience mental health problems than their peers, and children with learning disabilities, who were four times more likely than the general population to experience mental health difficulties. Additionally, 40 per cent of young offenders have a diagnosable mental health disorder. Overall, boys were found to be more likely to experience difficulties than girls, with 10 per cent of boys and 6 per cent of girls between the ages of 5 and 10 years having a mental health disorder, rising to 13 per cent and 10 per cent respectively for those between 10 and 15 years. Nearly 10 per cent of White children were identified with disorders, compared to 12 per cent of Black children, 8 per cent of Pakistani/Bangladeshi children and 4 per cent of Indian children.

Additionally, the children of lone parents are twice as likely to experience mental health difficulties (16 per cent compared to 8 per cent), and there was a higher prevalence in reconstituted families, where 15 per cent of children were affected. Risks of mental health difficulties were also seen to be higher in households with larger numbers of children and those where parents had no educational qualifications (15 per cent where parents had no qualifications, compared to 6 per cent of children where parent had degree-level qualification) or there was no working parent (20 per cent **prevalence**).

It is important, however, to consider that many of these categories are also likely to be associated with poverty, which is in itself associated with poor mental health (Wilkinson & Pickett, 2009). Additionally, when reviewing the evidence, it is relevant to consider that differences related to gender and ethnicity may also be affected by stereotypical expectations of behaviour and the extent to which these are embedded within assessments as well as access to culturally sensitive services. Furthermore, the association of poor child mental health with poor

Prevalence refers to the number of people having a condition at any one given time.

parental mental health found by Meltzer et al. (2000), and the finding that children with a mental disorder were more likely to have experienced several stressful life events, suggest that many children are growing up in a complex web of adverse experiences, including poor physical health, which cannot be easily unravelled or solved by any one intervention. It is also considered that such factors, in turn, expose children to more adverse experiences and that attention needs to be given to how children can develop resilience (Rutter & Smith, 1995; Rutter, 1999).

Bright Futures, a report commissioned by the Mental Health Foundation (Kay, 1999), based on a two-year inquiry into children's and young people's mental health, found that children are less likely to develop mental health problems if they have good communication skills, a sense of humour, religious faith, the capacity to reflect, at least one good parent–child relationship, affection, a family environment without severe discord, appropriate and consistent discipline and family support for education. Additionally, a wider support network within the community, good housing and living standards, a range of positive sport and leisure activities and a positive school environment offering strong academic and non-academic opportunities are also seen to be relevant factors in promoting positive mental health.

In the longer term there is evidence that mental health problems in children increase demands on personal social services, education, health and juvenile justice services, and are also costly for families. In a study of conduct disorder it was estimated that the lifetime costs in services used for individuals diagnosed with a conduct disorders at the age of 10 were over £100,000 more than for those without conduct disorders (Knapp & Scott, 1998).

The policy framework

Policy and guidance in this area are complex, but there are a number of themes and messages which are important in considering a mental health perspective when working with children and families.

The five key outcomes contained within *Every Child Matters* (Department for Education and Skills, 2004) provide the overall framework for children's services in England. The outcomes of being healthy, staying safe, enjoying and achieving, making a positive contribution and economic wellbeing clearly address overall health and wellbeing within a holistic approach.

The mental health and psychological wellbeing of children and families are specifically addressed in standard 9 of *The National Service Framework for Children, Young People and Maternity Services* (Department of Health, 2004c), where the need for timely access to integrated, high-quality, multidisciplinary services for assessment, treatment and support for children and young people experiencing mental health problems and disorders is emphasized. It is worth noting that

Tier	Professionals providing the service include	Function or service
Tier 1 A primary level of care	GPs Health visitors School nurses Social workers Teachers Juvenile justice workers Voluntary agencies Social services	CAMHS[a] at this level are provided by professionals working in universal services who are in a position to: • identify mental health problems early in their development • offer general advice • pursue opportunities for mental health promotion and prevention
Tier 2 A service provided by professionals relating to workers in primary care	Child and adolescent mental health workers Clinical child psychologists Paediatricians (especially community) Educational psychologists Child and adolescent psychiatrists Child and adolescent psychotherapists Community nurses or nurse specialists Family therapists	CAMHS[a] professionals should be able to offer: • training and consultation to other professionals (who might be within Tier 1) • consultation to professionals and families • outreach • assessment
Tier 3 A specialized service for more severe, complex or persistent disorders	Child and adolescent psychiatrists Clinical child psychologists Nurses (community or inpatient) Child psychotherapists	Services offer: • assessment and treatment • assessment for referrals to Tier 4 • contributions to the services, consultation and training at Tiers 1 and 2
Tier 4 Essential tertiary level services such as day units, highly specialized outpatient teams and inpatient units	Occupational therapists Speech and language therapists Art, music and drama therapists Family therapists	Child and adolescent inpatient units Secure forensic units Eating disorders units Specialist teams (e.g. for sexual abuse) Specialist teams for neuro-psychiatric problems

Figure 7.1   The four-tier strategic framework
[a] CAMHS = Children and Adolescent Mental Health Services
Source: Department of Health (2004c)

standards 6 and 7 also address the mental health needs of children and young people who are ill or in hospital.

The *National Service Framework* refers to the four-tier approach to mental health services for children and adolescents set out in Figure 7.1. Whilst the Children and Adolescent Mental Health Services (CAMHS) clearly have an important part to play in responding to the needs of children and young people experiencing mental health difficulties, it is significant that social workers and others are also seen as making a significant contribution, particularly in Tier 1.

More needs to be done to meet the needs of children from Black and minority ethnic communities, refugees and those seeking asylum, and continuing efforts are required to address long waiting lists and the lack of interpreters and to increase choice and involvement in referrals and preferred service location. There is also seen to be a 'serious inequity' (Department of Health, 2004c: 23) regarding access to services for children with learning disabilities and those at the upper end of the age range.

The increasing integration of children's services involving education, early years and social services is leading to new service models and a recognition that addressing the mental health needs of children needs to be incorporated throughout with both universal and targeted services. One example is the Targeted Mental Health for Schools Project initiated by the Department for Children, Schools and Families (2008) to improve the mental wellbeing of children aged between 5 and 13 years through a range of innovative and early interventions.

Drawing on these and other policies, it is possible to summarize the main themes as follows:

- co-ordinated services and integrated systems;
- interprofessional working;
- universal and targeted services;
- a holistic approach.

Whilst within this complex picture social workers may find themselves working in various service configurations and teams, these themes provide a sense of direction for practice, enabling social workers to recognize their contribution to the mental health of children and young people within a wider multiprofessional arena, stressing the importance of communication and co-ordination across a range of agencies and services.

Challenges of the early years

Whilst there is an emphasis on early identification and intervention where there are concerns about children's wellbeing, in reality difficulties in infancy and the early years are often challenging to identify and markers for positive mental health and wellbeing are hard to assess. The following discussion will briefly consider early infant development and the issue of attachment.

Early development: nature and nurture

There is increasing evidence regarding the impact of poor nutrition and physical care on early development. Findings reflecting a wide span of interdisciplinary research emphasize the complex interaction of genetic and environmental factors that takes place prenatally and early in life. A significant area of continuing research concerns the impact of early relationships on the development of the neurobiological structure of the infant brain and how this may affect later development:

> When the baby is born the brain is far from finished. Most of its neurons (about 100 billion) are present, but they are not part of functional networks. The prime task of brain development in the first few years of life is the forming, and then reinforcing into permanence, of necessary connections. (Balbernie, 2001: 239)

The term 'neuro-plasticity' is used to describe how the early development of the infant's brain responds to its environment, shifting previously polarized debates on the influence of nature or nurture on early development towards an interactive approach involving both, with Balbernie stating that 'The baby's eagerness to relate turns nurture into nature' (2001: 242).

Early experiences of 'good enough' parenting, including the provision of satisfactory physical and emotional care, assist the brain in the development of neural pathways that promote the potential for future learning, emotional resilience and the capacity for relationships based on sensitivity and empathy. In a paper examining the evidence for the impact of abuse and neglect on the development of the brain, Glaser (2001) refers to the 'neuro-biological' aspects of attachment and the way in which it may affect the baby's capacity to manage stress.

In less positive circumstances, Balbernie (2001) suggests that the experience of neglect or abuse may contribute to learning disability, language delay, lack of empathy, hyperactivity or poor impulse control. There may also be risks associated with the impact of maternal depression on infants between 6 and 18 months, which has been found to be associated with emotional and cognitive difficulties lasting until the start of school. It is also important to note that the biggest risk to development posed by Balbernie is in fact poverty, which may affect the quality of the physical environment and the nurture of the baby as well as impacting on the stress levels experienced by the baby's carers. The poor ranking of the UK on a number of dimensions of child wellbeing, including child poverty (UNICEF, 2007), indicates that this issue continues to be a priority.

Attachment

Attachment theory offers an important framework for understanding how young children make sense of their world. The concept is generally considered to have been developed by Bowlby (1979), whose work focused on the emotional bond that develops in the early relationship between the young child and their primary caregiver. This bond is demonstrated in attachment behaviour, which has been studied in terms of young children's responses to closeness and separation from their carer.

The concept is underpinned by the notion that infants are biologically primed to be attachment-seeking, in order for their basic needs, including food, shelter and protection, as well as affection and social relationships, to be met. For the majority of children, these early relationships are sufficiently warm, sensitive, consistent and reliable, leading to a sense of security. For others, however, a level of insecurity may result from care that is unpredictable, indifferent or hostile, leading to insecure or disorganized attachments that have the potential to influence relationships into adult life.

Undoubtedly other factors need to be considered in order even to begin to understand and assess the complexity of early child–caregiver relationships. However, Howe (2002) considers that attachment theory offers an example of a psychosocial perspective that can help in understanding social and emotional relationships both in childhood and in adult life. A focus on these early experiences also highlights the fundamental importance of safety and security, both emotionally and physically, in promoting future health and wellbeing.

This necessarily brief review of some highly complex material concerning early development draws our attention to some important issues. First, as is pointed out by Balbernie (2001) and Glaser (2001), it is vital that the potential to overcome early adversity is not overlooked and that although the early years are particularly significant in the development of neural pathways and connections, there is the potential for further development throughout life, assisted by a range of potential interventions including psychotherapy. Second, this discussion highlights the importance of supporting families before and after birth and through the early years. In the majority of situations this support is provided by other family members and within friendship and community networks. However, social workers and other professionals are in a key position to contribute in this area. Third, it may be helpful to consider the impacts of early life experience when working with adults experiencing mental health difficulties and to recognize the legacy of early difficulties.

This discussion also needs to be located within a wider perspective which recognizes differences of ethnicity and culture and a wider global perspective. Much of the literature discussed above is strongly rooted within a Eurocentric framework of understanding and experience and may not be easily transferable to different contexts where other priorities may take precedence. For children and families who are refugees or in war-affected countries, issues of trauma may arise in relation to dislocation or loss of home or close family members. In some parts of the world, high maternal mortality rates may lead to the disruption of early caretaking relationships. In other areas, limited access to clean water and lack of protection from diseases such as malaria may impact severely on physical development and wellbeing, with data from UNICEF (2008) indicating that 42 per cent of children under the age of 5 in South Asia and 28 per cent in sub-Saharan Africa are undernourished.

Reflection point

Amina left her home country after threats of violence and witnessing the torture of other family members. She has been granted refugee status after several years in Britain and has recently given birth to a baby girl. At times she has experienced periods of depression and says that she is socially isolated and has few friends. She tells you that her baby is very good and rarely cries. You have not seen Amina hold her baby although she clearly cares deeply about her.

Consider how you might talk with Amina about her baby's development and how she can increase her interaction.

In responding to the 'Reflection point' scenario, there may be a number of points that occur to you:

- You may be thinking that if Amina's baby is not causing any concerns, this is not a matter for you to consider, and to get involved might be seen as interference.
- You may be wishing to prioritize Amina's wellbeing rather than that of her child.
- At a more personal level you may find yourself reflecting on your own experiences of parenting within your family and considering the personal messages you have received about the care of infants.
- You may be aware that Amina's culture and background are unfamiliar and be wary of imposing your own views and knowledge.

It is important as social workers to think carefully about how, if and when to intervene in any given situation. However, in this example it may be possible to pay some attention to Amina's relationship with the baby. If you are confident about this – and not everyone is – you could ask to hold the baby and talk to and admire her, commenting positively on her response to being held and noting her interest in her surroundings. It might also be possible to emphasize Amina's capacity to care for her and to suggest that holding the baby might be pleasurable for both mother and baby. Notwithstanding any other ways of working in this situation, the development of this vital relationship can be encouraged in many different ways and can only hold benefits for the future wellbeing of both parent and child.

Common difficulties

Mental health problems in infancy and the early years may manifest themselves in difficulties in behaviour, which may be described by parents, carers or child care services, or in delays in reaching normal developmental milestones. Early attachment issues may also be spotted by health or early years services. However, as with all of these issues the child can only be assessed within a complex and holistic framework incorporating both their own and their carers' needs and experiences.

Interventions

A review commissioned by the Mental Health Foundation (Barnes & Freude-Lagevardi, 2003) examined a range of evidence regarding early interventions intended to enhance the mental health of young children and their families. The report concludes that interventions targeting both parents and children were found to be most effective, as were non-stigmatizing programmes that focused on disadvantaged and high-risk populations, building on strengths rather than deficits and addressing the psychological needs of parents, behavioural issues for both parents and children and social or situational stressors and supports. Feedback from practitioners highlighted the importance of shared decision-making with families and also emphasized a number of recommendations for interventions, which are summarized below:

- Nurture parents *and* children;
- Create the sense of a personal service by listening to people's stories;
- Start where the individual/family is, rather than where we think they should be;
- Keep in touch between appointments;
- Offer flexible and rapid access in family homes and with other professionals;
- Be prepared to give practical help before addressing parenting and child behaviour.   (Barnes & Freude-Lagevardi, 2003: 99)

Emphasizing the importance of early relationships, a Young Minds report concludes:

> The secure child is more likely to do well at school, form satisfying relationships, develop the capacity for compassion and empathy and have an inherent resilience in the face of misfortune. If we want more children to have a good start in life, one they will hand on to their own children, then the mental health needs of infants and their parents must be given the highest priority.   (Young Minds, 2004: 7)

The responsibility of social workers who have contact with parents and young children, regardless of their role and setting, is clear. However, it is worth noting that social workers and other early years professionals have been identified as being reluctant to consider the mental health of babies and young children, locating *mental health* within a deficit model of mental illness associated with particular symptoms and diagnosis rather than being associated with developmental well-being. Woodcock Ross et al. (2008) found that this reluctance to consider mental health was also associated with concerns about labelling and a focus on parenting styles and behaviour as opposed to a more interactive and relational approach which looked at the dynamic between parent and child. Such an approach has been viewed as leading to the marginalization of infant mental health needs within practice and to high thresholds of difficulties being required before interventions are considered.

> **Reflection point**
>
> Think back to the earlier example of Amina and her baby. Consider the extent to which you focused on either Amina's or her baby's needs. Were you thinking about Amina's parenting or the baby's behaviour as the 'problem'? Might there be any advantage in considering a more interactive approach?

In moving on to consider working with children who may be vulnerable to mental health difficulties, there can be a natural concern to avoid labelling due to concerns about stigma and discrimination that may ensue. There is also a tendency to be drawn to prioritize those situations where children are seen to be exhibiting behaviour that is troubling or challenging over those involving the quiet, withdrawn child. In the same way as mental health and illness may be 'constructed', it may be relevant to consider the social construction of childhood. For example, viewing children as 'innocents' may be accompanied by thinking that they are not affected by issues such as loss or other stressors, as they simply do not understand and therefore have no need to be supported in grieving or making sense of an unknown situation. Alternatively, as can be evidenced from the popular media, children's troublesome and challenging behaviour is sometimes framed as 'evil' and 'bad' rather than a demonstration of distress or confusion.

> **Reflection point**
>
> Think back to your own childhood or other experiences you may have of childhood. Can you identify any examples where your own or others' behaviour was framed in terms of a particular construction of childhood? Were there any particular attitudes or behaviours that were associated with this?

Whilst the activity in this 'Reflection point' might seem rather out of place in a book on mental health and social work, the intention is both to encourage the critical and reflective thinking that is central to social work and to highlight the different ways in which people make sense of different behaviour and situations. When thinking about issues of children's emotional wellbeing it is also necessary to be alert to issues of power and inequality in respect of the power differential that usually characterizes adult–child relationships.

One issue that may arise in response to this reflection is how issues of loss and death are handled within families. Sharing information about the loss of a family member or even a pet is often limited on the grounds that it is better not to upset a child or that 'they won't understand'. Attendance at a funeral may be ruled out, whether or not it would be appropriate for that individual child at that particular time.

There are likely to be many situations where the social worker is able to support parents in tackling sensitive issues with a child. This may be by encouraging them to explore their own fears about how the child might respond or by allowing them to recognize that it is their own distress that is the barrier. Recognizing the 'constructions' of childhood that may underpin their responses may help to offer alternatives in which children are viewed as active and thinking beings with their own views and feelings.

The 'Practice example' illustrates the potential involvement of social work in a complex situation, highlighting both the direct intervention and involvement in the wider system of services.

Practice example

David is 9 years old and lives with his mother, Sheila. His older half-sister, Natalie, is 20 and lives nearby. Sheila works part time and David often spends time with other family members after school, including Sheila's parents. David's father left the family five years ago and has only occasional contact. Sheila has experienced episodes of depression throughout her life and this has usually been treated by her GP with anti-depressant medication.

David initially settled at school, made friends and was seen to be making good progress. Over the last year his behaviour has changed and he has become unco-operative with the teacher and other pupils. Sheila has found that he is unwilling to play with his friends at weekends and prefers to watch television and play computer games. There have now been two recorded incidents at school where David was physically aggressive to other pupils and most recently he kicked his teacher when she tried to restrain him. A meeting has been called to discuss school exclusion.

Sheila discussed her worries about David when she visited her GP and he suggested that she talk to a social worker about the situation. Sheila reluctantly agreed as she did not want to be seen as an incompetent parent and was also worried about how social services might intervene, especially with her history of depression.

The social worker, Sunita, decides to meet initially with Sheila and also liaises with the school to let them know that she is involved. By chance Natalie is also present when she visits and takes part in the discussion about David after this has been agreed with Sheila. Sunita wants to make a full assessment as part of the Children's Assessment Framework (a standardized approach to undertaking assessment of children's needs; see Children's Workforce Development Council, 2009) and starts by asking Sheila to tell her all about David, not just the recent difficulties. She discovers that a year ago Natalie's boyfriend Pete was killed in a car accident. They had been seeing each other for several years and Pete had become close to all the family including David. They would play football together and sometimes Pete would take David to the cinema. Pete's sudden and unexpected death had been devastating for Natalie, and Sheila explained how she had had to provide her with a lot of support. Although David had been told that Pete had died, Sheila hadn't wanted to upset him too much, and David had been left in the care of his grand-parents for a number of weeks, often staying overnight at their home.

This 'Practice example' may also be considered in terms of the family model in Figure 7.2, which shows the interaction between three key areas, recognizing the influence of both risk and protective factors. This model highlights the interaction between the mental wellbeing of parents and children and the importance of a holistic approach when working with families. Additionally, the model emphasizes the need to take the strengths and resources of the family into account as well as any difficulties and problems they may be experiencing.

Reflection point

Consider how the family model in Figure 7.2 might assist you in the assessment of Sheila and David.
Does this also suggest ways of planning any intervention?

Having met with Sheila, Natalie and David, Sunita considers that it is likely that David's behaviour is a response to some of the difficulties that the family has been facing. There may be some particular vulnerability with Sheila being a lone parent as well as her experience of depression. The death of Pete represented a major loss for David and was also a stressor in terms of his own emotional wellbeing. Whilst well intentioned, the fact that David was sent away and not involved in Pete's funeral left him confused and distressed. Sunita's assessment is that overall this is a family that has a number of positive resources and that the fundamental parent–child relationship between Sheila and David is sound.

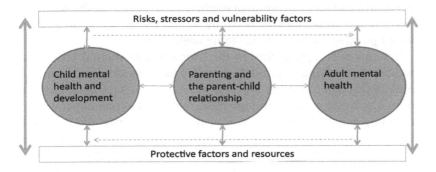

Figure 7.2 Family model
Source: SCIE (2009)

The forthcoming meeting to discuss David's exclusion from school creates some urgency in the situation as Sunita is anxious to look at the family situation overall, rather than simply focus on David. She is able to negotiate some planned sessions with Sheila on a time-limited basis in order to support her in responding to David's needs. At the meeting she is able to convince the school that she will monitor the situation and offer the teachers some time to discuss how best to manage David in the classroom setting. She is also able to refer David to an after-school group run by a school counsellor for children who are experiencing some difficulties.

Working with Young People

Adolescence is frequently seen as a period of 'storm and stress' as young people seek to establish their own identities and independence. Parents anticipate the teenage years with apprehension amidst an environment in which young people are often demonized in the media and political discourse. In reality the majority successfully navigate their way through with the support of families, friends and school, and it is only a minority of young people who are seen to be troubled and/or troublesome. At the same time there are some very real risks that signs of emotional and psychological distress may pass unnoticed or be subsumed within what is seen to be 'normal' adolescent development. Concerns from professionals regarding the risk of labelling young people may also divert attention from attending to potential mental health difficulties. The experience of mental ill health at this stage of life may disrupt developmental processes and transitions such as leaving school, further or higher education and employment, as well as the development of new social networks and a maturing sexuality.

It is important not to underestimate the challenges that are faced by young people as they mature physiologically, cognitively and socially, and to recognize that their ability to face these may also be affected by earlier life experiences and their response to adversity. Future research needs to focus on those young people who demonstrate the resilience to overcome difficulties successfully so that more can be understood about positive strategies to promote wellbeing.

Systems-wide approaches to the promotion of mental health and wellbeing involving communities and education services, from secondary through to further and higher education, have been found to offer a non-stigmatizing and universal approach to meeting the needs of young people, building self-esteem and confidence and a sense of social connectedness. Young people's familiarity with and access to the internet and mobile technology also offer opportunities. Such approaches benefit from co-operation between agencies and offer opportunities for social workers to contribute knowledge and expertise outside of an individual 'casework' role.

Significant variation between different individuals and groups of young people will also be found, reflecting different expectations based on gender, culture and community. Additionally, certain groups remain especially vulnerable and, as with the wider population, poverty, discrimination and disadvantage will affect the chances of developing a mental health difficulty.

Abuse and mental health

There is considerable evidence that childhood experience of abuse, both physical and sexual, may have longer-term consequences for mental health (Ackerman et al., 1998; Department of Health, 2002b; Spataro et al., 2004; Springer et al., 2007). A history of sexual abuse in both women and men has been associated with a twenty-fold increased risk of conduct disorders in childhood, an eight-fold increased risk of personality disorder and a five-fold increased risk of anxiety and acute stress disorders in adulthood (Spataro et al., 2004; Young et al., 2007).

It is also important to recognize that the responses to abuse will vary significantly between individuals and that abuse may be associated with other aspects of adversity. However, whilst not everyone who experiences abuse will go on to develop mental health or other psychological difficulties, it is clear that survivors of sexual abuse constitute a significant proportion of mental health service users, especially amongst women (Palmer et al., 1992; Mueser et al., 1998).

Plumb discusses the way in which the experience of abuse is characterized by being treated 'according to someone else's agenda' (2005: 112) and by feelings of powerlessness over what is happening. In turn this can lead to feelings of guilt, low self-esteem and lack of confidence, as well as depression, anxiety and post-traumatic stress disorder. In a survey of over 2,000 students, Martin et al. (2004) found that a sense of hopelessness contributed to 73 per cent of abused adolescents – compared to 25 per cent of those who had not been abused – having thoughts of killing themselves, with 45 per cent – compared to 9 per cent – claiming to have attempted to do so.

Looked-after children and young people

Children and young people who are 'looked after' are an especially vulnerable group in terms of mental health (Department of Health/ Department for Education and Skills, 2006: 37). Rates of mental disorder within this population are up to five times higher than for other children and young people, with 68 per cent of children living in residential care experiencing a mental health difficulty, often a conduct disorder, with a correspondingly increased rate of educational disadvantage and of being in trouble with the police (Office for National Statistics, 2003).

Practice example

Julie (aged 15) entered foster care three years ago following a child protection investigation as a result of her mother's alcohol and drug misuse. The breakdown of the foster placement led to Julie being placed in a residential unit where staff are increasingly struggling to manage her behaviour. Julie has threatened other residents and members of staff and attempted to harm herself on a number of occasions. She has also absconded and been returned by the police who found her on the streets late at night.

In considering the scenario in this 'Practice example', it may be useful to begin by recognizing the range of perspectives that may inform our understanding of the situation. As well as those of Julie herself and the residential workers, this is likely to include those of other agencies such as the police and education. Julie's mother or other family members may also contribute to the overall picture. In reviewing the situation, Julie's social worker will also be drawing on her or his own knowledge, values and experience.

Reflection point

What are the factors that may be affecting Julie's behaviour?
   To what extent is it helpful to consider this scenario in terms of Julie's mental health?
   What might be helpful in responding to the situation and how, as Julie's social worker, could you support her in voicing her own concerns and wishes?

Although the limited information available here allows only a level of speculation about the factors affecting Julie's behaviour, it is relevant to acknowledge the potential impact of her experiences before and after entering care and the way in which these various transitions have been managed. Additionally, whilst there might be a reluctance to label Julie's behaviour, she would appear to be demonstrating a level of distress that demands a response, although opinions may differ as to what this should be. There is also a need to consider her safety, as well as that of others, as a major priority. It is not unlikely that she will be experiencing a level of powerlessness about her situation and it will be important for her views to be listened to and acknowledged by someone she can trust and who can advocate for her.

Although this scenario may or may not be seen as a 'mental health' situation, there are clearly elements of mental wellbeing at stake which may be highly significant for Julie's future, and the involvement of CAMHS or other opportunities for therapeutic work may be helpful. The provision of support and information for other workers and agencies may also assist them in continuing to work with Julie.

Self-harm

Self-harm includes self-poisoning and self-injury such as cutting behaviour and is most common in those under the age of 25 years, especially young women. In one school survey (Hawton et al., 2002) it was estimated that girls were three times more likely than boys to self-harm, with 13 per cent of young people between the ages of 15 and 16 claiming to have self-harmed at some time in the past and 7 per cent in the previous year.

It is widely recognized that life events including victimization, sexual abuse and relationship difficulties are strongly associated with self-harming behaviour, and hence self-harming needs to be seen as a marker for the presence of other problems (Meltzer et al., 2002; National Institute for Health and Clinical Excellence, 2004). Certain groups are seen as especially vulnerable, including lesbian, gay and bisexual young people as well as young people in residential settings and young Asian women (King & McKeown, 2003; Bhugra et al., 1999).

Eating disorders

It is estimated that 2 per cent of all women experience some form of eating distress, and this is likely to begin at an early age, with the average age of onset for **anorexia nervosa** and **bulimia nervosa** being 15 and 18 years respectively. One survey found that 31 per cent of 15-year-old girls were dieting, leading to an eight times greater risk of developing an eating disorder than for non-dieters (Patton et al., 1990). Although much of the attention in this area has focused on the needs of young women, there is also growing concern regarding young men and eating disorders.

Young carers

Children and young people involved in caring for someone with a mental health difficulty, usually a parent, comprise one third of all young carers, of whom there are an estimated 175,000, although the true figure may be higher as young people taking on this role are often hidden or not defined as carers. Over 15 per cent of young carers are from minority ethnic groups and overall it is suggested that girls and young women are more likely to be involved in caring for their mothers (Roberts et al., 2008). Whilst it is important not to paint an overwhelmingly negative picture of young carers' experiences, evidence suggests that they may be disadvantaged in terms of their education and social relationships as well as affected by the stigma associated with mental illness. On the positive side, many children and young people take a pride in supporting their parents (Cooklin, 2006) and make an important contribution to domestic tasks and providing practical and emotional support.

Anorexia nervosa a condition where someone is very concerned about being overweight and will eat very little, regardless of their actual size. Control over weight loss and body shape may be seen as a positive achievement, despite others' concerns.

Bulimia nervosa a condition involving binge eating and the use of laxatives and/or vomiting as well as excessive exercising to control weight. This behaviour may be managed in secret and changes in weight may not be noticeable. Both anorexia and bulimia can have severe health consequences and may be life-threatening.

Recognizing the presence and needs of young carers is the first step towards accessing the support that may be available, often through specialized services that may be provided by statutory and non-statutory organizations working in partnership.

Concluding Comments

This chapter has drawn attention to the importance of an integrated approach to thinking about the needs of families. In particular, there is a need to 'bridge the gap' between social work practice with children and families and social work practice with adults experiencing mental health difficulties. A 'think child, think parent, think family' approach has been presented, promoting a more joined-up approach to working with parents with mental health difficulties and encouraging greater communication and co-ordination between mental health and children's services.

Social work offers many opportunities to promote emotional well-being and resilience for children and young people and their carers. These may often be addressed most successfully by supporting parents or others in recognizing and responding to the needs of children and young people in their care. Being aware of the needs of children and young people who may be especially vulnerable to mental health difficulties will help to ensure that appropriate resources and interventions are made available for individuals and, more widely, to support mental health and wellbeing.

Further Reading

SCIE (2009) *Think Child, Think Parent, Think Family: A Guide to Parental Mental Health and Child Welfare.* London: SCIE

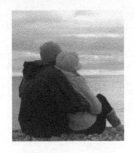

8 The Mental Health Needs of Older People

Key points

- The impact of ageing and ageism on mental health in later life
- Recognizing and responding to depression among older people
- Working with people with dementia
- Older people as carers

Introduction

Setting arbitrary boundaries on the basis of age could appear to run counter to social work principles of respect for the individual and the importance of challenging discriminatory practices. At the same time it is important to identify some of the experiences that may be shared by those at a certain point in their lives, not least the impact of ageism. This provides a frame of reference for considering later life and a lens through which the social, emotional and physical aspects of ageing can be viewed and understood. The rationale for this chapter is to ensure that attention is paid to social work practice with older people and the many opportunities this may create to address aspects of their mental health.

Foregrounding age and in particular later life, as in this chapter, also has its limitations. Arbitrary markers of age in terms of years do not always reflect reality, such as the younger person with a diagnosis of early-onset dementia or a person in their seventies unable to access psychological therapies, crisis resolution or assertive outreach services that are restricted to those under 65 (Healthcare Commission, 2009). In terms of critical practice, it is also valuable to reflect on the consequences of the drawing of boundaries that are set up to address the practical realities of service organization and delivery. Such distinctions often demonstrate the limitations of dichotomous thinking – the example here being the arbitrary distinction between young and old – that, if accepted uncritically, have the potential to limit the benefits of any intervention.

However, focusing on life course may also be relevant when considering the organizational patterns and structures which frame much of social work practice in the UK and where work with children and families is distinguished from work with adults, which in turn is frequently still separated from work with older adults.

Reflection point

Consider from your own experience any situation where arbitrary boundaries on the basis of age
have limited access to services.
   Can you suggest any more creative solutions to this way of organizing services?

In addition to acknowledging the importance of a trajectory through
life and the potential cumulative effect of different experiences over
time, it is also important to recognize the interaction at any one time
of biological, psychological and social factors. Attention will be paid to
a number of these issues in the discussion that follows in this chapter.

The Policy Framework

As in the previous chapter, where the social construction of childhood
was briefly explored, it is relevant here to consider the social construction of ageing and to acknowledge the sometimes negative connotations associated with becoming older. Despite demographic changes
and increasing longevity leading, for example, to changes in arbitrary
notions of retirement age, the institutionalization of old age continues,
located within social and political structures and supported by discriminatory attitudes and practices. Within mental health this has
been manifest in the cut-off for many services at 65 and a preoccupation with dementia rather than a wider approach to mental health and
wellbeing. Very often services for older people are seen as 'Cinderella'
services, poorly resourced and staffed by low-paid workers with limited
access to training. More generally Llewellyn et al. refer to the 'tendency
to see the over-65 age group as an homogenous group with similar
needs, leading to a one-size-fits-all model of service provision' (2008:
231). Changes in social care policy and provision point to the continuation of the tensions that lie beneath approaches to older people's
mental health and wellbeing, with a number of policy documents
setting out to address the mental health needs of older people alongside the range of policy and guidance that applies to the mental health
of adults of any age.

   The *National Service Framework for Older People* makes the clear
statement that 'services will be provided, regardless of age, on the basis
of clinical need alone' (Department of Health, 2001b: 12). Mental
health is addressed within Standard 7, the aim of which is to promote
good mental health in older people and to treat and support those
older people with dementia and depression.

   The mental health needs of older people also feature in the *New
Horizons* document (Department of Health/HM Government, 2009)
with regard to improving the recognition and treatment of depression
as well as early intervention in dementia. These are, however, seen as

additional approaches to meet the particular needs of older adults, alongside the broader range of services and interventions offered to adults of any age.

In practice, the proliferation of policy and guidance has created some confusion as to how these should be interpreted. For example, in older people's services the introduction of the Single Assessment Process (SAP) and plans for a Common Assessment Framework intersect with the Care Programme Approach (CPA) for mental health services. Department of Health guidance (2004b) states that where an older person is assessed as having a psychotic condition their needs should be assessed under the SAP but their care should be managed by the CPA. Where other mental health problems are identified, both the assessment of need and care management should be undertaken within the SAP. In the case of people reaching the age of 65 who have been receiving mental health services, there is no need to transfer from the CPA to the SAP. Additional difficulties may be experienced by the social worker who is employed within the local authority and subject to local authority systems whilst working with a community mental health team where health systems predominate. There may also be tensions between health and social care regarding the funding of services. The absence of integrated IT systems may be a further barrier to joined-up working. Such confusion can be overcome with effective communication and co-ordination between workers and teams, although breakdown of systems is frequently associated with people falling between services, with sometimes tragic consequences. More frequently, media attention is drawn to the distress caused by delays in accessing services, problems of 'bed-blocking' and the gap between health and social services. A report by the Healthcare Commission (2009) on older people's mental health services points to the lack of a 'standard model of care' and suggests that 'The ways in which we divide organisations and services in policy, planning, implementation and regulation can potentially deprioritise an area such as older people's mental health' (2009: 7). In the midst of this somewhat confusing picture it is important to hold on to the principles of person-centred care summarized in Figure 8.1.

The development of the Positive Opportunities for Older People programme (POPPS) prioritized new and joined-up ways of thinking about mental health and wellbeing, with nineteen projects across England. These were intended to develop more integrated services to address mental ill health, offer preventative interventions and promote social inclusion, with activities including dementia cafés, the provision of talking therapies and walking or gardening groups. Some of these were specifically planned to target Black and minority and lesbian and gay communities (Department of Health, 2005). However, longer-term budgetary constraints and political debates regarding the future of public spending on care services may limit the effectiveness of such initiatives. The emphasis on welfare-to-work policies and

Maintaining the person's sense of wellbeing and promoting their personhood

Recognizing the life experience and unique biographies of individuals

Maintaining social networks, family, previous interests and life histories

Seeing the *person* – not the diagnosis

Nurturing respect, dignity and self-worth

Focusing on the person's remaining abilities, with no-failure strategies [i.e. every

opportunity is taken to maximize the chance of success]

Using affection, empathy and warmth in our work

Figure 8.1 Principles of person-centred care
Source: Minshull (n.d.)

changes in the social security system which emphasize the importance of employment for people with mental or physical ill health, whilst beneficial for many, at the same time highlights an approach which values people for their productivity and economic contribution and thereby perpetuates a view of ageing that implies deficit and dependency.

Mental Health Difficulties in Older People

When considering mental health in older people there is frequently an assumption that this primarily concerns the development of dementia. However, figures suggest that whilst about 5 per cent of the population over 65 has dementia, about 10–15 per cent of the population over 65 will experience depression. The risk of dementia does nevertheless increase with age, leading to an incidence of 20 per cent over the age of 80, affecting 600,000 people in the UK (Department of Health, 2001b).

It also important to recognize that dementia and depression may well occur together, with the symptoms of early dementia themselves increasing the risk of depression as someone finds themselves less capable of managing independently and maintaining activities which previously contributed to their quality of life. There is also the risk that the symptoms of depression may be mistaken for dementia. Regardless of diagnosis and age, mental health difficulties in older people need to be understood within the context of their life experiences and as part of unique, individual narratives, reflecting the opportunities, adversities and disadvantage which continue to influence and impact on mental health and wellbeing. Additionally, these will be influenced by the experiences of increasing physical ill health or disability and the loss of partner, family and friends, which together may impact both on the availability of social networks and on the ability to maintain these.

Dementias

As already indicated, dementia affects increasing numbers of people as they become older, although it is relevant to note the incidence of early-onset dementia and the particular difficulties this may generate, both for the individual concerned and for their family and friends.

Various types of dementia have been identified, with the most commonly occurring being Alzheimer's disease. This affects 50–60 per cent of people diagnosed with dementia, with vascular dementia and dementia with Lewy bodies (similar to Parkinson's disease and characterized by hallucinations and falls) each affecting 10–15 per cent (McKeith & Fairburn, 2001). These would all be understood as organic conditions where evidence of the disease process can be identified in the brain, although this is normally only detectable after death in Alzheimer's. The causes of Alzheimer's are as yet undetermined, although vascular dementia is understood to result from damage to the blood supply in the brain related to small strokes or thromboses. In some other dementias there is evidence of a genetic component, whilst, for example, Korsokoff's syndrome is related to a history of high levels of alcohol use.

Early indicators of Alzheimer's include poor recollection of recent events and difficulties in absorbing new information or dealing with new situations. Everyday activities may become difficult and there may be a level of paranoia as the person tries to make sense of the changes they are experiencing. Insight is intermittent and cognitive impairment may affect thought and communication. As the condition develops, carers and neighbours may become concerned about night-time wandering and the individual's increasing inability to care for themselves. The person may at times become distressed or anxious and it may become difficult for carers to reassure them. Later on, personality changes may become evident and incontinence may develop.

Although there is no cure for any of the dementias, there is widespread agreement that early diagnosis is desirable and a range of support can be offered. For Alzheimer's, drug treatments such as donepezil (Aricept) may be effective in slowing the disease process in its early stages in 40 per cent of the people treated. This treatment is not licensed for any other form of dementia and is only recommended for people with mild to moderate Alzheimer's, as determined by the **mini mental state examination (MMSE)** (National Institute for Health and Clinical Excellence/Social Care Institute for Excellence, 2006). An initial comprehensive assessment and treatment should always involve specialist services, although ongoing care may be shared with the GP, with drug treatments continuing only if there is no deterioration and

Mini mental state examination (MMSE) a brief screening test for cognitive impairment.

MMSE scores remain above 10. Anti-psychotic drugs are also sometimes used to treat psychotic symptoms, although atypical drugs can increase the risk of stroke. A report by the Audit Commission (2000) also recommends that a full assessment of physical health is undertaken and that attention is paid to any accompanying depression.

Increasingly, social workers are employed in specialist mental health teams which aim to offer a holistic response to both the person affected and their family and carers. The quotation below offers an important reminder about the need to see beyond the diagnosis:

> If we view dementia only as a 'disease', then we are tempted to abdicate our fundamental responsibility as human beings for the welfare of our fellows, and leave it to scientists in laboratories to discover the pill, potion, gene or magic bullet that will 'treat' or even cure dementia. But if we see dementia as a condition of which organic degenerative brain disorder is only one part, but which is also fuelled by the fear, anxiety, shame and incomprehension of both the person concerned, those who they are in contact with and the wider society – then we can begin to see that we have a role to play ourselves.
>
> (Barnett, 2000: 24)

The work of Kitwood (1997) has been particularly influential in the shift from an emphasis on dementia as a disease to an understanding based on psychological and social as well as biological perspectives. His Enriched Model of dementia is closely allied to notions of personhood which he saw as being undermined by 'Malignant Social Psychology', including experiences of being infantilized, disempowered, objectified, ignored and stigmatized. He recognized that Malignant Social Psychology, whilst unintentional in many situations, can become institutionalized within dementia care practices. The development of Dementia Care Mapping by Kitwood and others involved in the Bradford Dementia group (1997) offers an approach to measuring the person-centredness of a care environment based on the experiences of those with dementia, and has been used to support and monitor the process of change. The approach is not without its difficulties; however, an increasing evidence base is seen to support its continued development (Brooker, 2005).

The elements of person-centred care have also been identified by Brooker (2007: 13) as:

V   A value base that asserts the absolute value of all human lives regardless of age or cognitive ability.
I   An individualised approach, recognising uniqueness.
P   Understanding the world from the perspective of the service user.
S   Providing a social environment that supports psychological needs.

Such an approach can be seen as central to opposing discrimination and promoting social justice in social work. Parsons (2005) highlights how social workers are able to work within a rehabilitative frame to maintain quality of life for people experiencing dementia and their carers across a range of service settings and teams, recognizing that assessments and commissioning of services within a broad care management role offer a unique opportunity to offer a social perspective. The training of social workers, and others, as Best Interest Assessors also offers opportunities to contribute to the resolution of complex and delicate situations balancing risk, freedom and dignity.

There are particular challenges for social work in this area. Workers may often find themselves acting as intermediaries between carers requiring more support, such as night sitters, and the insufficient resources that may be on offer. Issues of hope and recovery that underpin approaches to mental health difficulties earlier in life may be hard to maintain, and notions of choice and self-determination may require determination and creativity to ensure that the voice of the person is heard.

The 'Practice example' introduces Jack, a 78-year-old man, and Rose, a social worker from an Adult Care Team.

Practice example

Jack is 78 and has lived alone since his wife died three years ago. Until recently he appeared to be managing on his daughter, but his son, who visits every few weeks, is beginning to have some concerns about how her father is coping. Jack has always been fiercely independent and still insists that he doesn't need any help. However, it appears that he has lost weight and on a recent visit his daughter found that there was no sign of Jack preparing meals or eating regularly. When asked about what he was eating, Jack became defensive and said that it was difficult to do this when people kept interfering. When pressed, Jack was unable to tell his daughter any more about who was interfering and how.

Jack's daughter has also contacted the team to ask for advice about finding a residential home. At the same time one of Jack's neighbours has called the police to report that Jack has frequently been found standing outside their house looking in through the window but refuses to say what he is doing.

Having read the story so far, think about the way in which you might begin to make an assessment of Jack and your response to the following questions:

- Who would you want to talk to, to find out more about the situation?
- What kind of information would you want to find out?
- Are there any particular issues you would want to keep in mind when meeting Jack?

In some respects, it would be easy to see this as a straightforward request for information from Jack's daughter, although there is the added complication of the police involvement, as they have also contacted the service after attempting to visit Jack, who was unwilling to open the door when they called. Rose, the social worker allocated to respond to the initial referral, decides that there is sufficient concern to assess the situation using the SAP, but in the first instance decides to talk to Jack's daughter to explain how this works and also to provide her with information about referrals for care homes, pointing out that this might be one of a number of options that would be appropriate. In her experience she has found that family members are often unaware of how older people can be helped to maintain their independence at home and may also need support in recognizing that it is the person themselves, as far as is possible, who needs to make any decisions about their future care. Meeting Jack's daughter will offer Rose the opportunity to find out more about the family and their involvement with Jack. Rose also contacts Jack's GP for more information.

In planning to visit Jack, Rose is aware from the information she has so far that Jack may be very anxious about a visitor, especially with his recent experience with the police. She decides to write to Jack but also asks if his daughter can be present for the first part of their meeting, as she thinks that this may help her across the threshold. Rose suspects that Jack is not aware that he has been referred and she wants to make sure that, from now on, Jack is fully in the picture. Depending on how the visit unfolds, Rose is mindful that she may need to talk to the neighbours, with Jack's consent, and also involve his GP, possibly by suggesting he make an appointment for a general check-up.

In thinking about her meeting with Jack, Rose is aware that it will be important not to overwhelm him with too much information and to ensure, as far as possible, that there are minimal distractions, such as the TV. She has found that simply slowing herself down before meeting someone, taking a few deep breaths and trying to relax, however busy or stressed she might be, helps to tune in to someone who may be frightened or bewildered by what is going on. This will also assist her in listening and observing in order to build up a comprehensive picture of the situation.

When she first arrives at Jack's home and introduces herself to Jack and his daughter, Rose is struck by how able he appears. Jack welcomes her into the house and asks her to sit down, asking what 'all this' is about. Before Rose can answer, however, his manner changes, and he asks if she can help him to find his wallet as someone has moved it again. In response to her question as to who might have moved it, he looks out of the window at his neighbour's house and says that he can't say. Rose takes this opportunity to suggest that they have a look for it together and Jack agrees to this, allowing Rose to be shown into the kitchen, where it appears that there is little in the cupboards and the fridge is virtually empty.

In reflecting on her visit to Jack, Rose feels reasonably confident that she has gained a good deal of information about the situation and that she has established a good rapport with Jack, although it will be important to re-establish this relationship again next time she visits, as she is unsure of how much he will remember. She is pleased that Jack and his daughter have agreed to make an appointment with the GP, as she suspects that Jack is in the early stages of dementia and she knows that Jack's GP is positive about the benefits of early diagnosis. The issue of residential care was not raised at the meeting and Rose thinks that Jack's daughter is less anxious about this now that an assessment is under way.

More immediately, Rose has identified two issues that, having discussed them with Jack, she can address straightaway that may help the situation. First, she will attend to a referral for the Home Support team in Jack's area and request that he be assessed for support that could include help with shopping and meal preparation. Second, having discovered Jack's interest in music, she will contact the local community centre, where a music group for older people takes place, to see if Jack might be able to join.

Rose is aware that, if she is correct in thinking that Jack has early dementia, a more intensive support plan will be required. However, she is confident that a full assessment using the SAP and a comprehensive care plan, carefully worked out with Jack, will enable her and others to support his independence and wellbeing for as long as possible.

Depression

At the time of writing, 2.4 million people over the age of 65 experience depression, and this is expected to rise to 3.1 million by 2021. However, depression in older people is frequently unacknowledged, and research suggests that only a third of older people with depression discuss it with their GP, and of those only half are diagnosed and receive treatment (Mental Health Foundation, 2009).

Depression may also be taken for early dementia, given the presence of confusion or poor memory. However, in depression these may fluctuate over time whereas with dementia they are likely to increase in both frequency and magnitude. Self-reported concern about confusion or memory is more likely to be associated with depression than with dementia. Depression may be indicated by changes in levels of physical activity, either a reduction or an increase, accompanied by agitation and distress, by feelings of guilt and worthlessness and by disturbed or changed sleeping and/or eating patterns.

Other conditions may also be relevant to consider in relation to older people's mental health. Some of these may be related to the presence of physical health difficulties, which may significantly impact on wellbeing, both directly and indirectly. Infections, including urinary tract infections, may cause confusion, or a fall causing a broken wrist, the diagnosis of heart disease or diabetes may contribute to a sense of decreasing independence and increasing vulnerability. Older people may also be more vulnerable to adverse drug reactions, particularly when a number of different medicines are prescribed. Such reactions may in themselves disrupt eating and sleeping patterns in addition to more severe reactions, leading, for example, to a toxic confusional state, delusions or delirium. Psychological trauma associated with a heart attack or serious injury, or with assault or burglary, may also need to be recognized and addressed.

Ray and Phillips (2002) refer to the need to develop what they term 'gerontological social work' based on critical practice, the importance of challenging pathological and ageist assumptions, tackling inequalities and disadvantage and working towards empowerment. These will be illustrated in the 'Practice exmple' concerning Glenda, which will also highlight the importance of engagement and communication in working with older people experiencing mental health difficulties.

Practice example

Glenda was born in Barbados and in the 1960s moved with her husband to England, where they settled and had three children. Another child was born in Barbados and brought up by Glenda's mother after she had moved away. Glenda has visited only a few times, most recently for her father's funeral six years ago.

Glenda's husband, Errol, died suddenly two years ago. Before his death they had been planning their retirement and had intended to return to Barbados. Glenda has worked for most of her life but gave this up after Errol's death. It was at about this time that her two daughters left home, one to get married and the other to work in another part of the country. Until recently Glenda has been an active member of the local church, where she has been involved for many years.

Two weeks ago Glenda didn't attend a local church meeting and when visited by a friend was found sitting at home. She appeared dishevelled and unable to talk, becoming tearful when questioned by her friend. Her youngest child, who lives at home, explained that she hadn't left the house for several days, didn't seem to be eating and hadn't been to bed for at least a week. He could think of no explanation for his mother's behaviour although he did say that she had recently heard from his sister in Barbados, who was unwell.

He also reported that she had been waking very early and seemed to have lost interest in life.

Glenda's behaviour caused her friend to call Glenda's GP, who visited briefly and said that he would refer Glenda to the local community mental health team for older people.

Consider that you are the social worker who is asked to visit Glenda. How might you assess this situation?

Yasmin, the social worker who is allocated this referral, is immediately aware of the need to respond urgently as the referral indicates that Glenda's physical health may be at risk if she is refusing food and drink. At the same time, the information Yasmin has received suggests that the situation will require attention to other important aspects of Glenda's life. Yasmin is also mindful of the comments of one of her colleagues, who says that this referral could quickly turn into a Mental Health Act assessment.

The approach requires practitioners to: 1. Examine the situations they encounter with service users from the individual's perspective as well as their own 2. Weigh up options for intervening including the value base underpinning practice and the practice context together with their own practice experience 3. Make an informed judgement that is acted upon 4. Reflect on the outcome of their action/decision-making 5. Critically appraise what they have learned

Figure 8.2 Five-stage approach to mental health social work practice
Source: Bailey (2002: 170)

Yasmin draws on Bailey's (2002) five-stage approach to mental health social work practice as she has previously found this to be helpful in responding to complex situations such as this. Bailey suggests that this approach assists mental health social workers to be clear about their roles within multidisciplinary settings, recognizing the various strands of professional accountability and responsibility. The five stages are set out in Figure 8.2 and build on the basic key roles including assessment, planning, intervention and evaluation.

On arriving at Glenda's home, Yasmin is greeted by Glenda's son, Stephen, who is clearly very worried about his mother. He takes her into the kitchen where Glenda is sitting, seemingly unaware of anyone around her. Yasmin gently resists Stephen's attempt to draw her into the hall to talk privately and instead sits down next to Glenda, introducing herself and suggesting that Glenda appears to have a lot of upsetting thoughts on her mind. She asks if Glenda would be prepared to tell her about some of these, and after sitting in silence for some time, Glenda says flatly that 'it's too late'.

With encouragement from Yasmin, Glenda talks a little more about her family and nods when Yasmin asks if she would like her to get her a drink. Yasmin also talks about how other people are concerned for Glenda's wellbeing and that whilst life clearly feels very difficult for her at present, there is every chance that she will feel better in the future.

Yasmin also involves Stephen in the discussion at this point and stresses to them both how important it is for Glenda to drink and eat to avoid becoming dehydrated. Yasmin is concerned to avoid the trauma of hospital admission if at all possible, although equally aware that this may be necessary if Glenda is not able to respond quickly. Before leaving she arranges to call again the next day.

Reflecting on her visit, Yasmin feels that she has been able to begin to build a picture from Glenda's own perspective and that there is the potential for further work with Glenda to address her experiences of change and loss. Yasmin is also reasonably confident that Glenda is not yet at the point of requiring urgent medical care, although she is aware that the situation requires careful and regular monitoring and that she needs to retain an open mind.

In terms of options for intervention, Yasmin is anxious to maintain Glenda's independence and involvement in her care. She is particularly aware that the risks of Glenda's physical health deteriorating could lead to hospital admission, possibly under the Mental Health Act, and that it would be preferable to avoid this if at all possible. Yasmin is also aware that Glenda, as an older Black woman, is likely to have experienced discrimination in her life and that Black Caribbean women are at greater risk of compulsory detention under the Mental Health Act (Care Quality Commission, 2010). At the same time, it is important that Glenda receives appropriate care and support and, as Yasmin begins the formal assessment process, she considers the resources that might be available. Her judgement is that these include Glenda's existing resources within her own family and community as well as her own strengths and experiences. The main points of the plan that Yasmin draws together are as follows:

- Make a referral to a community-based counselling service, with Glenda's consent.
- Provide Glenda with information on depression.
- Talk with colleagues about the possible benefits of medication.
- Assess the needs of Glenda's son as a carer.
- Develop a crisis plan in case the situation deteriorates.

Reflecting on her initial assessment and plan, Yasmin feels confident that this can be presented back to her team. This will need to be accompanied by a risk assessment and Yasmin recognizes that she will also need to consider how support can be offered to the family, especially Stephen, as the main carer. Yasmin considers too how important it is for her to maintain her social work perspective and values within the multidisciplinary team where the pressure of work and concerns about risk can quickly take precedence.

This scenario also offers the opportunity to reflect on the issues that might arise if Glenda were assessed as in urgent need of inpatient care and she were either unable or unwilling to consent to admission or treatment. Previous discussion in Chapter 4 highlights some of the complexities associated with the use of the 2007 Mental Health and 2005 Mental Capacity Acts, and the reader may wish to revisit these in the light of this 'Practice example', recognizing the role of advocacy in contributing to the protection of human rights.

Other Aspects of Social Work Practice

The following 'Practice example' brings us back to Rose, a social worker in an inner-city Adult Care Team, and highlights the importance of thinking about mental health in communities as well as at an individual level.

Practice example

Rose has received a number of referrals from Home Care, Sheltered Housing and the local Health Centre concerning older people who are isolated and living alone, frequently with a range of health and mobility problems. She is aware of the high level of depression experienced by older people and how this risk may be increased by social isolation.

When Rose discusses her caseload in supervision she suggests setting up a group where people could offer one another support. However, her manager is concerned that the focus of the referrals was on an assessment of physical needs and that this work has now been completed. Furthermore he questions issues of confidentiality if Rose were to go ahead with this plan.

Rose decides to talk to other colleagues in the team about this to see if she can gain any support for her idea. One colleague suggests that they make contact with a neighbourhood network for older people in the local community. Over a lunchtime meeting an agreement is reached to explore the possibility of joint working to set up a support group. A further meeting is arranged with a plan to invite some of the older people themselves who are already known to be interested.

This example provides an illustration of a number of relevant issues for social work practice. In identifying an area of need, Rose and her colleagues are drawing on their own knowledge and experiences gained from working in the local area, as well as wider research regarding older people's mental health and the effects of social isolation. A second issue concerns the pressures of practice and the perspective of the team manager, who may be under pressure to meet certain targets and to 'contain' any work that does not address these. However, the conversation that follows with her colleagues and the suggestion of contacting the voluntary sector group opens up another perspective, offering the potential for a collaborative initiative.

The involvement of representatives from the local group at an early stage also emphasizes the benefits of participation and avoiding the risk of making assumptions about what might be best for a group of older people. It will be important, however, in this example to consider how the interests and needs of diverse groups of older people might be represented, rather than simply responding to the voices of those who are already active in the local community.

In terms of responding to inequalities, there may be the potential for a more active campaigning group than Rose had initially envisaged. Other agencies are already aware of the impact of poor public transport and a lack of meeting places in the local area, and this may be seen as contributing to the high levels of social isolation and depression amongst older people there.

It is relevant to remember that many older people are carers themselves. Although the carers in the practice examples offered in this chapter were the daughter and son respectively of Jack and Glenda, there are many situations where the main carer is the partner, sibling or friend of the older person with mental health difficulties. Figures suggest that 15 per cent of the over 65s are carers and that overall, 24 per cent of carers are over 65 (NHS Information Centre, 2010). In total it is estimated that 1.5 million people over the age of 60 years are providing unpaid care, of whom 8,000 are over 80 (Buckner & Yeandle, 2005). Whilst women make up the majority of carers overall, carers over the age of 65 are more likely to be men.

This raises important considerations for social work practice, recognizing the potential impact of caring on the health, wellbeing and finances of the carers themselves (Carers UK, 2007). Individual carer's assessments accompanied by information and support are vital, and there is potential for close working with other agencies in the statutory and voluntary sectors to address the needs of carers through community-based initiatives. Dementia cafés offer a positive example of the way in which support can be offered to people with dementia and to their carers, combating social isolation, promoting peer support and providing information and signposting to other resources (National Mental Health Development Unit, n.d.).

Concluding Comments

Practice in this area may offer particular challenges for social work. First, these may relate to working in an environment where issues of policy, service configuration and resourcing for older people with mental health problems may be contested and contradictory, resulting in 'buck-passing' between different agencies. Second, social workers are likely to find themselves located at the nexus of competing demands from carers and other service providers, whilst attempting to foreground the wishes and needs of the individual older person. There may be different and conflicting views about what is and isn't acceptable in terms of risk and managing uncertainty. All of this is underpinned by ageist attitudes and values in which older people are often denied a voice, respect and dignity and are deemed incapable by those around them.

The contribution of social work with an emphasis on anti-oppressive practice is particularly important when working with older people, including the responsibility to challenge negative attitudes and misinformation, for example regarding the widely held view that memory loss is inevitable with increasing age. Social workers may also need to consider their own views and behaviour, which may reflect the experience of traditional social work caseloads. These inevitably present a high proportion of older people who are experiencing difficulties, rather than representing a wider spread of the population, and create only a partial perspective on older people's lives.

Despite criticisms that social work education is often accused of failing to prioritize work with older people and mental health issues in general, reflecting the double jeopardy effect experienced by service users as both old and having poor mental health, the knowledge, skills and values associated with social work remain the fundamental bedrock of practice in this area.

Further Reading

Mental Health Foundation (2009) *All Things Being Equal: Age Equality in Mental Health Care for Older People in England.* London: Mental Health Foundation

Resources

Mental Health in Later Life: www.mhilli.org
Dementia gateway: getting to know the person with dementia. Available at www.scie.org.uk/publications/dementia/know/getting. asp, accessed 13 November 2009

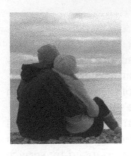

9 Working with People Experiencing Depression, Trauma and Other Difficulties

Key points

- Recognizing and responding to depression and anxiety
- Dual diagnosis, alcohol and drug use
- Working with people diagnosed with a personality disorder
- Mental health associated with physical health difficulties
- The contribution of cognitive behavioural therapy
- Responding to disaster, trauma and abuse and their impact on mental health
- The need for social workers to take care of themselves

Introduction

This chapter will focus on social work practice with adults who are experiencing mood disorders including depression and anxiety, as well as other mental health difficulties not generally involving psychosis. Reference will be made to the association of mental health difficulties with alcohol or drug abuse, working with people with a diagnosis of personality disorder, and mental health difficulties that may be experienced by people with physical health problems. The use of cognitive behavioural therapy will be discussed, as will the impact on mental health of trauma, abuse and violence, including domestic abuse.

An important message from this chapter is that social workers may encounter people experiencing these difficulties in a number of different situations. In some cases, mental health issues may feature clearly in an initial referral, whilst in others, mental health considerations may emerge during the assessment phase of social work contact. Social workers may also become involved in responding to the needs of families, groups and communities who may be experiencing mental health difficulties in response to particular events or circumstances such as natural disasters.

This chapter also highlights the need for social workers to take care of themselves and to acknowledge their own personal responses when working alongside people who are depressed or distressed. Talking issues through in supervision or seeking out support, especially if feeling stressed or burnt out, are an essential part of being a professionally competent social worker.

The Impact of Depression and Anxiety

When compared with other conditions, such as an episode of psychosis or a diagnosis of schizophrenia, there can be a tendency for depression and anxiety to be viewed as less serious and less deserving of attention. However, the impact of depression or anxiety on the quality of life of many individuals and their families can be long-term and seriously disabling. Internationally, it is recognized that whilst depression is ranked as the seventh most important cause of disease burden in low- and middle-income countries, it can often remain untreated. For women, there are also clear links with reproductive health and the impact of gender on access to socio-economic resources and status, and issues of abuse and violence. Additionally, depression in women is linked to lower rates of breast feeding and higher rates of postnatal depression, potentially affecting early relationships and child development (WHO, 2009a).

Despite declining rates of suicide in men and women across all age groups in the general population, it is relevant to note that depression is associated with a higher risk of suicide. The *Annual Report: England and Wales* of the National Confidential Inquiry into Suicide and Homicide by People with Mental Illness indicates that among people in contact with mental health services, those with **affective** disorders, including depression, continue to have the highest suicide rate when compared to other diagnoses(National Confidential Inquiry, 2009a).

Affective a term used to refer to the emotional component of psychological distress.

Wilkins refers to the 'paradox' that men are three times more likely than women to take their own lives but only half as likely to be diagnosed with depression (2010: 33). However, there is increasing recognition that the incidence of depression amongst men may be higher than previously thought, due in part to the ways in which men's emotional wellbeing is understood, recognized and recorded (Royal College of Psychiatrists, 1998; Wilkins, 2010). It is suggested that men may be more likely to demonstrate their distress with anger or that it may be masked by alcohol or drug use. In turn, these responses have the potential to obscure recognition of any underlying depression and to act as a barrier to accessing help and support.

Within families, children may be affected by a parent experiencing depression, which may impact on parenting style. Depression in fathers may increase the chances of a child developing a depressive illness in later life, while depression in mothers may also impact on the child's relationship with their father (Parrott et al., 2008).

The mental health of older people and their access to appropriate services are explored more fully in Chapter 8. There are widespread concerns that high rates of depression in older people, whether they are living in their own homes or in residential care, are not adequately identified or addressed (Department of Health/HM Government, 2009; Mental Health Foundation, 2009).

Reflection point

To what extent are social workers more likely to identify depression or anxiety amongst women than amongst men? Is there anything that social workers could do differently to address men's mental health needs?

You may find it helpful to refer back to Chapter 6 when considering these questions.

The wider costs of depression can also be measured in financial terms. Newspaper headlines refer to the costs to the economy of people not working because of depression, estimated at £8.6 billion in 2009 (*Independent*, 16 July 2009). Such figures exclude the costs of health care for depression, including visits to GPs, estimated as £33 million in 2007–8, and medication, estimated at £264.5 million. In Britain, it is estimated that one in five GP consultations are about common mental disorders, and mixed anxiety and depression is estimated to cause one fifth of days lost from work (McManus et al., 2009). Evidence such as this can be seen to have been influential in the development of new policies and services intended to promote mental well-being and to offer new treatments.

It is important, however, to be cautious about the extent to which such discussions emphasize a negative discourse of 'burden' when such data is publicized. Pilgrim (2009) points out that, whilst legitimate in many ways, such debates fail to acknowledge the positive contributions that may be made by people experiencing such difficulties in terms of creativity, caring for others or involvement in services.

Depression

To be diagnosed with depression requires more than feeling miserable or down. In addition to depressed mood, tiredness and fatigue, and a loss of interest or enjoyment, a number of other features may also be present. The following form part of the ICD-10 (International Classification of Diseases, tenth iteration) classification of Depressive Episode (WHO, 2007):

- reduced concentration and attention;
- reduced self-esteem and self-confidence;
- ideas of guilt and unworthiness;
- bleak and pessimistic views of the future;
- ideas or acts of self-harm or suicide;
- disturbed sleep, including early morning waking;
- diminished appetite and weight loss;
- loss of libido.

Diurnal variation patterns of change throughout the day.

ICD-10 notes that there may be little change from day to day although there may be some **diurnal variation**, with symptoms being most severe in the morning. These indicators must usually be seen to be present for at least two weeks before a diagnosis is made.

For depression as for other diagnoses, a number of different explanations have been put forward. These include the influence of biological factors on the biochemical balance in the brain, which feature particularly in discussions of bipolar disorder, where depression may be accompanied by periods of **mania** and there is some evidence of a genetic predisposition. The contribution of hormonal factors is also recognized in certain forms of depression, as is the effect of an underactive thyroid, both of which can be successfully treated if recognized. There is also now greater acknowledgement of Seasonal Affective Disorder (SAD), understood as resulting from the impact on the brain of changing levels of sunlight through the year.

Cognitive models of depression focus on core beliefs and the associated negative thinking that may result from early experiences and stressful life events. Seligman (1975) proposed that 'learning' that one is unable to control events can lead to a sense of 'learned helplessness' that contributes to the development of depression. Early work undertaken by Brown and Harris (1978) drew attention to the social causes of depression amongst working-class women, paving the way for further work in this field. At the heart of each of these explanations is the notion that depression stands as a valid diagnosis and a medical condition that is amenable to various forms of treatment.

Alternatively, the concept of depression has been challenged as a diagnosis and instead understood as an existential or spiritual experience. Such approaches are rooted in the notion that sadness is an inevitable part of human experience and an understandable response to life events. There are also concerns that the concept of depression is not universally recognized and that experiences and emotions may be manifest in many different ways, depending on culture and context. For example, within Chinese culture, an ethic of hard work and perseverance may make it particularly challenging when someone displays the tiredness, lack of interest and motivation associated with depression, leading to conflict between family members and delays in seeking help. Additionally, a holistic understanding of the mind and body in traditional Chinese medicine have led to a high level of **somatization** in the way in which emotional difficulties are presented (Yeung, 2003).

Treatment for depression includes:

- *Medication*: Anti-depressant medication is recommended in severe depression although not seen to be appropriate for mild depression, where any benefits may be outweighed by negative side effects and there is a chance that the depression may resolve without treatment. Where anti-depressants are prescribed they may take several weeks to take effect, and this is important to note where the risk of suicide may be a concern. Lithium carbonate is a mood-stabilizing drug

Mania a state of high arousal, agitation and restlessness associated with bipolar disorder. For some people mania may also be related to periods of creativity.

Somatization the experience of psychological distress being understood and explained in terms of physical symptoms.

that is used to treat bipolar disorder, requiring careful monitoring to maintain the appropriate therapeutic level.

- *Psychological treatments*: A range of 'talking therapies' may be offered, including interpersonal psychotherapy or counselling. Cognitive behavioural therapy (CBT) is increasingly being made available, sometimes in conjunction with medication. A more detailed discussion of CBT will be found later in this chapter.
- *Electroconvulsive therapy (ECT)*: ECT involves passing an electrical current through electrodes attached to the head, in order to induce a small seizure. A number of treatments may be given over several weeks. This is only likely to be offered in severe cases where the impact of depression may be life threatening in terms of suicidal intent or an inability to eat or drink. The use of ECT remains controversial. Its use for older people has been justified in terms of their limited tolerance of anti-depressant medication, but this has also been challenged on the grounds that older people, and older women in particular, are offered fewer treatment alternatives, especially with regard to psychological interventions.

The contribution of social work to working with people with depression

It is particularly relevant for social workers to be mindful of the various ways in which depression may be understood and to consider how they can respond to people experiencing loss, bereavement, family breakdown, physical illness or disability, which may also be accompanied by feelings of sadness and helplessness.

One woman describes her experience of depression as follows:

> I can remember particularly bad days. I would only take the day in 10 minute chunks because that was it. I couldn't bear to think oh I've got all day at home here not feeling like I can do anything, yet feeling bored and feeling bad about myself. And thinking all these negative thoughts all the time. Everything in my head was negative. And that I couldn't feel anything for [husband]. I couldn't feel anything for the children. It was like being inside a very, very thick balloon and no matter how hard I pushed out, the momentum of the skin of the balloon would just push me back in.   (Healthtalkonline, n.d.)

Whilst each situation will require its own unique response, the skills that may come to mind are likely to include both active and non-

Activity

Read or watch a first-hand account of the experience of depression and consider how you might respond as a social worker if someone were to share experiences of this kind with you.
  What social work skills would be important in how you might do this?
  What effect might this have on you at a more personal level?

selective listening skills, empathy and the sensitive demonstration of assessment skills, using open questions to explore further details of the experiences of the service user and their situation (Trevithick, 2007). Sometimes simply sitting in silence alongside someone who is distressed, however hard this may be, in itself can convey respect, positive regard and empathy. Non-verbal communication skills, requiring attention to body language, eye contact, posture, physical proximity and expression, are important elements to consider, as well as the choice of language used, the tone and the quality of empathic responses. The use of physical touch requires very careful consideration and can run the risk of being inappropriate or misinterpreted.

Much will depend, of course, on any pre-existing relationship and the extent to which a level of trust and safety has already been established. The physical context in which the encounter takes place will also impact on the way in which the worker is able to respond. Sitting in a 'safe' space in a private office or someone's home may feel very different from a meeting involving other workers, the presence of children or other family members, or a conversation over coffee in a public space. Many social workers have experience of highly sensitive discussions taking place in their cars whilst driving. Whilst there may be a level of psychological safety in such situations, it is of course essential to reconcile this with the need for physical safety, and it may be necessary to negotiate and plan for further time to talk when full attention can be given.

The reality of practice is that social workers can often feel under considerable pressure to 'do something' when faced with someone in distress. This tendency can be fuelled by heavy workloads and organizational demands to meet deadlines and targets. Equally, this can be a normal and understandable response at a more personal level to distract attention from the difficult feelings that may arise in a situation of this kind. This is where access to regular supervision can be invaluable in providing a safe environment to examine your own emotional feelings and responses. It is important to be able to acknowledge and reflect on how these may affect practice and, where appropriate, to feel able to seek out support or develop strategies for promoting personal mental wellbeing.

The 'Practice example' demonstrates the need for a sensitive social work response to a carer who is experiencing depression as his partner, with early-onset dementia, is being offered respite care in a residential home.

Practice example

Sean has early-onset dementia, and Mike and Eddie have been attending a care planning meeting held at the residential home where Sean is staying. Mike has been the main carer for Sean for the past three years and has reached a point where he is not sure that he can continue to look after Sean at home. Until recently this has felt manageable with the support of friends and some professional care that he has been able to afford from a private organization, with Mike continuing to work part time.

The social worker involved, Eddie, has met Mike before and found him to be very much in control and clear about accessing appropriate services and support for Sean. However, on this occasion, Mike seems tense and Eddie observes that he looks tired and stressed. When Eddie asks him how he is coping, Mike becomes very upset. For a number of minutes Eddie sits quietly with Mike and simply acknowledges how difficult things must have been, commenting that it is not surprising that Mike feels so distressed under the circumstances.

Slowly Mike begins to talk about how things have been for him over recent months. He tells Eddie that he has felt very alone and isolated, as many of their mutual friends live some distance away and it has become increasingly hard to keep in touch. Relationships with both of their families had been difficult at times, and although information about local support groups for people caring for someone with early dementia had been offered to Mike, his one attempt to make contact had caused some discomfort when it became clear that he and Sean were gay.

Mike also talks about not sleeping and losing weight as well as feeling very negative and despondent about the future, as he and Sean had had so many plans. He expresses some guilt that he is not able to continue caring for Sean at home and is anxious that he will feel responsible for any further deterioration in Sean's condition. He also comments that it is self-indulgent to ask for help for himself in comparison with Sean's needs.

Eddie realizes that there will be no quick fix to enable Mike to feel better, but that it will be important to think about the situation using a psychosocial perspective. He is aware that Mike has bottled up his feelings for a long time and that some aspects of the situation require sensitivity to the needs of Mike as a gay man. He plans to meet with Mike again very soon to assess further how he is coping and allow him time to talk. Eddie considers suggesting that Mike visits his GP, which might also offer access to some short-term counselling. Eddie has also heard of a lesbian and gay support network run by the Alzeimer's Society, and thinks this might be a useful contact for Mike.

Later, reflecting on his meeting with Mike, Eddie realizes that he was himself quite distressed by the situation and asks himself how much he was affected by witnessing another man being so upset in addition to the other challenges involved. He notes that this could be something to raise in supervision.

Anxiety and other related conditions

Within conventional systems of diagnosis informed by the ICD and the Diagnostic and Statistical Manual (DSM), anxiety is seen as falling into one of the following types:

- phobic anxiety disorder including agoraphobia;
- panic disorder;
- anxiety disorder;
- obsessive-compulsive disorder.

As with depression, when considering anxiety, we find that in addition to the standard indicators which make up the ICD-10 classification, there are wider debates concerning the associated underlying emotions and causes which might generally be seen as linked to fear. Within a psychoanalytical approach, there is an emphasis on understanding anxiety as unresolved conflicts relating to early development and experience, whilst for the behaviourists, anxiety is seen as a response to a fearful situation. A social perspective locates anxiety and fear within a wider social context, recognizing issues of power and inequality.

One of the distressing components of anxiety is the accompanying physiological sensations such as palpitations, breathlessness or nausea, as the person experiencing them may fear that they are having a heart attack or be about to collapse physically, feeding into a vicious circle of anxiety. Such experiences can be seen as part of a fight-or-flight response which is also a survival mechanism, reminding us that anxiety can serve a valuable and protective purpose in the face of a threat.

Phobic disorders are associated with fear in response to a specific event or experience, such as enclosed spaces or spiders. This can be extremely disabling and in some circumstances may leave someone unable to leave their home, with significant consequences for everyday life and social relationships.

Obsessive-compulsive disorders (OCDs) may include both a cognitive and a behavioural element, with the obsessional thoughts, for instance, relating to a fear of dirt or contamination, and associated compulsive behaviours intended to relieve the fearful thoughts. Whilst it is not unusual for many of us to 'double check' whether or not we have locked the door or turned off the iron when we leave the house, OCD can result in the repetition of checking, cleaning or handwashing rituals which come to dominate the individual's life and severely affect the lives of those around them.

Treatment for this group of difficulties is frequently behavioural or cognitive behavioural therapy and may include **desensitization** programmes for phobic disorders. The association of anxiety and depression may also lead to the use of anti-depressant medication. Referral for social work involvement may arise when difficulties are long-term and the condition has had a major impact on the life of the individual and their family, requiring strategies for rebuilding social networks and activities as well as specific interventions to address the condition itself.

Desensitization a process involving the gradual exposure to the thing or situation that is feared. A desensitization programme is carefully tailored to the individual and will include developing strategies for managing the fear.

Mental Health, Alcohol and Drug Use

There is a complex relationship between mental health and the use of alcohol or other substances, with 80 per cent of people receiving treatment for alcohol misuse experiencing anxiety and depression, and up to 50 per cent of those with mental health problems misusing alcohol or drugs (Department of Health, 2009a). However, it can be difficult to unravel the precise association, recognizing that alcohol or drugs may be used as a self-medicating strategy for managing depression, or may contribute to or exacerbate depression, or both. Indeed, attempting to clarify 'what comes first' may divert attention from the real issues involved and contribute to people being excluded from services (Crome et al., 2009). There are also particular issues regarding the relationship between psychosis and cannabis use, and these will be referred to in Chapter 10.

Dual diagnosis describes the simultaneous presence of two conditions. The term is frequently used when mental health difficulties and alcohol or substance use occur together, but may also be used when an individual is seen as having a learning disability and a mental health problem.

The term **dual diagnosis** may be used in different ways, but is frequently applied where a mental health difficulty is accompanied by alcohol or substance misuse. For service users and carers, the experience of dual diagnosis can include the risk of being passed between services and falling through the gaps, despite the acknowledgement that people with a dual diagnosis are likely to have more severe mental health difficulties and increased risks of suicide, violence or victimization, and are less likely to comply with medication or treatment. Additionally, they are more likely to be involved in the criminal justice system and to have a history of sexual or physical abuse in childhood (Watson & Hawkings, 2007). At the same time the range of agencies that may be involved in providing services creates a complex picture of provision, although there is now a clear policy statement that care should be mainstreamed within mental health supported by collaborative working between different services (Department of Health, 2002a).

The development of alcohol treatment pathways (ATPs) has the aim of ensuring 'the right people, doing the right things, in the right order at the right time, with the right outcome, right first time – all with attention to the service user's experience and allowing for comparison of the planned care with the care that was actually delivered' (Department of Health, 2009a: 4). Social work involvement in this area may arise as a result of joint working between specialist alcohol services and mental health teams where assessments, undertaken either separately or independently, are used to develop shared care plans, which are jointly implemented and monitored with close attention to liaison and communication between the agencies involved (Department of Health, 2009a). The association of dual diagnosis with homelessness (Department of Health, 2002a: 9) may also lead to opportunities for social work involvement.

A briefing by the Social Care Institute for Excellence (Crome et al., 2009) suggests that co-existing mental health and substance use problems may affect between 30 and 70 per cent of people presenting to health and social care settings. The report also highlights the limited research undertaken from a social work or care perspective, despite the high risk of self-harm and suicide and the likelihood that social exclusion and social problems will be present. There are, however, clear messages regarding the importance of person-centred and non-judgemental approaches in developing supportive relationships, working to build on strengths rather than pathology and undertaking holistic assessments which take into account the individual's own story. It is important to avoid making stereotypical assumptions which may obscure the recognition of alcohol or substance use in older or younger people, women and those from ethnic minority groups, as well as to ensure that interventions are sensitive to issues of difference.

Personality Disorders

An alternative to the conventional definition of personality disorder set out in Chapter 2 is offered below:

> not an illness you catch or are born with, but ... a 'way of being' you develop while growing up. It means some aspects of your personality cause repeated problems in life – particularly with relationships. The troubled relationships can be with family and friends, work and care services – and frequently with all of them.
>
> (National Personality Disorder Programme, n.d.)

The emphasis on troubled relationships contained in this definition captures some of the challenges involved in working with people who are seen to have a personality disorder, as such difficulties are an inherent part of the problems for which they are seeking help, as well as being an obstacle to seeking and accepting that help.

It is estimated that up to 13 per cent of the population may be affected by personality disorder, with potentially higher levels in deprived urban areas and amongst the homeless, the prison population and those with other forms of mental health difficulty. Although the formal diagnosis refers to ten sub-types of personality disorder, two forms – anti-social personality disorder (ASPD) and borderline personality disorder (BPD) – are most commonly encountered by social workers and other health and social care professionals.

People with ASPDs often exhibit 'traits of impulsivity, anger and associated behaviours including irresponsibility, recklessness and deceitfulness. They have often grown up in fractured families in which parental conflict is typical and parenting is harsh and inconsistent' (National Institute for Health and Clinical Excellence, 2010). Borderline personality disorder is often associated with the experience of trauma or abuse in childhood and may be characterized by the following symptoms:

- having emotions that are up and down;
- feelings of emptiness and anger;
- difficulty in making and maintaining relationships;
- having an unstable sense of identity;
- self-harm.

> (National Institute for Health and Clinical Excellence, 2009a)

It is recognized that women are more likely to be diagnosed with BPD whilst men, particularly in the forensic and criminal justice systems, feature more prominently with ASPD (National Personality Disorder Programme, n.d.). Although a diagnosis of personality disorder is not usually made before the age of 18, ASPD is seen to be associated with conduct disorders in childhood, and early interventions with families are recommended (National Institute for Health and Clinical Excellence, 2010). It is of interest to note that the guidance on BPD (National Institute for Health and Clinical Excellence, 2009a) does refer to the incidence of BPD amongst young people, and acknowledges the potential risks of intervention, including the reinforcement of problematic behaviours as well as the dangers of undertaking trauma therapy in a young person who may be vulnerable to impulsive behaviour.

Increasing attention and resources are now being channelled towards this area of work, and various forms of therapy, including cognitive therapy, dialectical behavioural therapy and therapeutic community approaches, are seen as offering positive ways forward.

Self-referral and choice in accessing services based on promoting hope and optimism are seen to be essential. The need for workers who can build trusting, consistent and reliable relationships, whilst maintaining clear boundaries, is also recognized.

Further discussion of working with personality disorders can be found in Chapter 11, where activities based on the case study of Mervyn will be used to illustrate issues of risk and risk assessment within a context of interprofessional working. To some extent, however, locating this discussion within a chapter on risk is an issue of practicality and should not preclude the recognition of people with relationship difficulties amongst those with other mental health issues.

Mental Health Conditions Associated with Physical Conditions or Disability

Social workers working with people with physical illness or disability often find that they need to respond to mental health issues which may be either directly or indirectly associated with the particular condition. The complex interrelationship of physical and mental health and the need for a holistic approach are also illustrated by the fact that depression is experienced by 20 per cent of people with a long-term physical health problem – two to three times more than among those in good health (National Institute for Health and Clinical Excellence, 2009a). For example, depression is a high risk factor for coronary disease, whilst of those people who have an acute heart event 20 per cent will have a major depressive episode within a few weeks, and a third of those with congestive heart failure have depressive symptoms. Whilst it is possible that there may some biological factors involved, the presence of depression can also have a negative impact on the way in which individuals respond to treatment and aftercare, potentially leading to poorer outcomes in terms of physical recovery or overall quality of life (British Heart Foundation, 2005).

Liaison psychiatry departments within general hospitals work to bridge the gap between psychiatry and medicine for individuals experiencing complex physical and mental health conditions. For social workers, the use of a bio-psycho-social model may also help in acknowledging the various factors which may require attention in terms of assessment and intervention, as in the 'Practice example'.

Practice example

Audrey is 56 and was diagnosed with multiple sclerosis (MS) fifteen years ago. Until two years ago she worked in the accounts department of a telephone company, but she took early retirement when her health deteriorated. Leaving work meant that she became less active and she lost contact with a number of friends. She was also increasingly affected by fatigue, seen to be related to her MS. However, the social worker, George, who was asked to see her was aware that 50 per cent of people with MS may experience depression at some point and wondered whether Audrey's tiredness was also an indicator of depression, or could even be partly contributing to her depression, as Audrey was becoming increasingly frustrated by her limited energy and inability to maintain previous levels of activity. Additionally, he was concerned that changes in Audrey's medication might be affecting her energy levels.

Through the process of undertaking a collaborative assessment with Audrey, George began to build a more detailed picture of her life. This included recognizing the effects of disappointments and setbacks as a result of her MS as well as having to live with the uncertainty of a relapsing condition. Drawing on a social model of disability, George and Audrey were able to explore the impact of the diagnosis on her relationships and her sense of exclusion from a range of social activities, recognizing that this had also affected her self-esteem and self-confidence.

George recognized that it would be important for Audrey to feel empowered in tackling some of her difficulties. They planned how she could talk with her consultant about her medication and the side effects, resulting in a useful discussion and some modification to her treatment.

Audrey also talked about her feelings of being useless, which had increased since she had retired. Adopting a solution-focused approach, George encouraged her to imagine how things could be different. This led to Audrey setting herself some realistic goals for the future, recognizing the need to be flexible in response to the uncertainty of her condition.

Cognitive Behavioural Therapy

Cognitive behavioural therapy (CBT) is based on the premise that what you think affects how you feel and what you do, and sets out to intervene in this cycle by tackling the relationship between thoughts, feelings and behaviours. Unlike some other therapies, the primary focus of CBT is in the 'here and now', rather than searching for the origins of difficulties in previous experiences, although these may be considered if they are relevant. The main emphasis is on addressing the situation as it is in the present and identifying strategies for change.

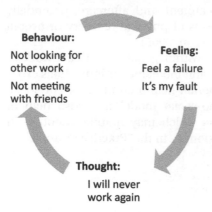

Figure 9.1   The relationship between thoughts, feelings and behaviours

Based on a systematic approach to assessment and treatment, CBT addresses the vicious circle that may develop between thoughts, feelings and behaviour, as illustrated in the simple example in Figure 9.1, which might result from being made redundant or becoming unemployed.

Cognitive behavioural therapists emphasize the importance of establishing a positive therapeutic alliance and using a collaborative approach in their work. Problems and goals are clearly identified and a case formulation is drawn up to help make sense of the difficulties and how these link to the thoughts, feelings and behaviours involved, as well as to related events and experiences. This then provides a collaborative rationale for the therapeutic work and helps to create a clear agenda for each session. Homework may also feature, such as keeping a diary or record of events, thoughts and feelings or trying out new behaviours as 'experiments'.

CBT case formulations can be developed at different levels of complexity, beginning with the automatic thoughts that are relatively easy to access and, for experienced therapists, moving into a deeper exploration of underlying assumptions and core beliefs. Certain forms of CBT may be offered by means of self-help manuals, computerized or not, some of which have accompanying worksheets and guidance for practitioners.

Social work and CBT

In the UK, CBT has been endorsed by the National Institute for Health and Clinical Excellence (2009b) as the preferred treatment for people with depressive symptoms or a diagnosis of mild to moderate depression (and anxiety) and forms a central element of the Improving Access to Psychological Therapies (IAPT) programme. For people experiencing more severe depression, CBT or interpersonal therapy accompanied by anti-depressant medication is recommended. A stepped model of care offers a range of interventions from low to high intensity, depending on the severity of the condition.

The emphasis on CBT, however, is not without its criticisms, including the view that CBT is a 'quick fix' and not likely to address longer-term and more deep-seated difficulties that may underlie depression (Leader, 2008). The IAPT agenda is also closely aligned with a political and economic agenda concerned with reducing absence from work and the costs of sickness benefits. Additionally, there are concerns that disproportionate weight is being placed on the evidence base for CBT, as opposed to other forms of therapy which have been less extensively researched, and that overall the evidence remains inconclusive (Roth & Fonagy, 2004). Objections to CBT include concerns that the approach could be manipulative or unethical, with the potential for changing behaviour in response to crude behaviour modification techniques. Advocates of CBT counter this by emphasizing the importance of negotiation and collaboration in agreeing both the overall goals within therapy and the means of achieving them.

From a social work perspective, CBT has been seen as failing to recognize the impact on mental health of wider factors such as oppression and discrimination although there is a growing recognition of such issues (Levinson, 2010). It is interesting to note that whilst CBT may not be high on the list of social work approaches, other more popular interventions, such as solution-focused therapy and task-centred social work, can be seen as having similarities with CBT in their emphasis on goal setting, tasks and activities with clear time scales for review and endings.

Activity

Look at a range of information available on the internet regarding the use of CBT for people experiencing mental health difficulties.

Consider the situations where you think this might be appropriate in terms of your role as a social worker with a service user experiencing depression.

What might be the benefits of CBT?

When might it not seem appropriate?

Cigno, a social work advocate of CBT, argues that:

> attention to both the immediate and wider environment and their tradition of intervention in the client's own home setting put [social workers] ... in an ideal position for developing applications of cognitive-behavioural theory to the real and often untidy, oppressive world of clients of social welfare in local authority and other non-clinical settings.
>
> (2002: 181)

Trauma and Abuse

Regardless of setting, it is not unusual for social workers to encounter situations where individuals have experienced various forms of trauma, either recently or in the past, that continue to impact on their daily lives. Sometimes these issues may be treated as a 'hot potato' and quickly passed on to another agency. Alternatively, they may be ignored or overlooked as too challenging to identify and address explicitly.

Whilst it is important not to assume that everyone who has experienced abuse will go on to develop mental health difficulties, evidence suggests that there is an association between child sexual abuse and self-harm, depression and anxiety as well as eating disorders and drug and alcohol abuse. Domestic violence, most of which is perpetrated by men on women, is estimated as being experienced by between 18 per cent and 30 per cent of women in their lifetime. Women experiencing domestic violence are also more likely than other women to report depression and make greater use of mental health services (Department of Health, 2002b).

A study undertaken for Women's Aid (Barron, 2004), in relation to women's mental health and domestic violence, found that questions about experiences of violence or abuse were not routinely asked and that mental health professionals lacked training and confidence in tackling the subject. Workers were sometimes reluctant to open up issues, especially where these were not seen as the key agency priority and might in themselves cause further distress.

It is vital that experiences of abuse or violence are not overlooked or dismissed in people who have experience of mental health difficulties. There is also a need for more training for staff and services offering specific interventions and support for people who have experienced violence and abuse.

Reflection point

As a social worker, how might you raise issues of violence and abuse when working with people experiencing mental health difficulties?

Identify the knowledge, skills and values that would help you to do this sensitively and constructively.

Post-traumatic stress disorder

Post-traumatic stress disorder (PTSD) is defined by the World Health Organization as 'a delayed or protracted response to a stressful event or situation (either short or long-lasting) of an exceptionally threatening or long-lasting nature, which is likely to cause pervasive distress in almost anyone' (WHO, 1992: 147). The diagnosis of PTSD was added to the DSM in 1980. However, the psychological and emotional impact of trauma and stress had been identified for many years across a range of situations, including the 'shell shock' of First World War veterans and the experiences of survivors of fires and natural disasters. PTSD is also caused by domestic violence or sexual abuse and experiences of torture (frequently related to civil unrest and in those seeking asylum). There is need for caution, however, in noting that although 30 per cent of people experiencing a traumatic event may go on to develop PTSD, many will not, although both groups may benefit from support (National Institute for Health and Clinical Excellence, 2005).

A central feature of the traumatic situation is seen to be its exceptional and threatening nature, and a response characterized by feelings of powerlessness and helplessness. Herman (1992: 33) writes that 'at the moment of trauma, the victim is rendered helpless by overwhelming force ... Traumatic events overwhelm the ordinary systems of care that give people a sense of control, connection and meaning.' From a global perspective the application of the diagnosis of PTSD is not without its difficulties, particularly in resource-poor countries dealing with war, civil conflict or disaster. The concept has been challenged for its medicalization of distress that can be seen as a normal and understandable response to a threatening situation, and as a further demonstration of the application of models of illness developed within the Western world which may not be recognized as cross-culturally valid or relevant in other health care systems (Bracken et al., 1995; van Ommeren et al., 2005).

The main 'symptoms' associated with PTSD include the following:

* avoidance of reminders of the situation, which may include people, places or talking or thinking about the event;
* numbing or lack of feeling, which may extend to other parts of the person's life and include feelings of detachment from other people;
* re-experiencing the situation in flashbacks or nightmares;
* increased arousal with exaggerated startle responses (for example, responding to everyday sights and sounds as if they are threatening), irritability, sleep problems and difficulties in concentration.

Depression, drug or alcohol abuse, anger or unexplained physical symptoms may also be present in someone with PTSD.

In the immediate aftermath of a traumatic experience, guidance for England and Wales recommends a four-week period of 'watchful waiting' without routinely offering individual debriefing where symptoms are mild (National Institute for Health and Clinical Excellence, 2005). Specialist trauma-focused treatment is recommended for those with severe difficulties.

Children can develop PTSD and this may require careful assessment to ensure that appropriate interventions and support are offered to all members of the family. Signs of distress in children may include nightmares, social withdrawal and regression to previous behaviours, such as clinginess or bed-wetting, although these may resolve over time without professional intervention. The role of social workers in such situations is often to focus on supporting parents and carers who are best placed to respond to their children's needs.

Social work responses to communities affected by trauma or disaster

Although social work may have a part to play in responding to disasters both nationally and internationally, it is important to acknowledge that communities and individuals possess their own processes for survival and recovery. As well as emphasizing principles of human rights, equity and participation, the Inter-Agency Standing Committee (IASC) suggests that 'stand-alone services are rarely sustainable, generate stigma and fragment already splintered care systems' (Inter-Agency Standing Committee, Reference Group on Mental Health and Psychosocial Support, 2010: 5). Attention has also been drawn to the need for social workers and others to work at the community as well as the individual level to offer responses that take into account wider social, political and cultural issues. Examples of community-based responses include work in Northern Ireland to promote community cohesion and peace-building (Piachaud, 2008) as well as women's collective responses to sexual violence in Uganda (Bracken et al., 1995).

Working with individuals, families and communities whose lives have been affected by trauma, abuse or disaster is likely to be challenging and potentially stressful for all involved. It may also be a natural response to look elsewhere, outside of social work, for specialist knowledge and skills. Some of these undoubtedly exist and are of value. However, it is as important to return to and draw upon fundamental social work values and knowledge, which continue to provide a clear framework for practice in this area.

Harrison and Melville (2010) refer to a resurgence of interest in human rights and social justice in social work, partly fuelled by the work of the International Federation of Social Work, although there are continuing concerns that this remains primarily at the level of academic discourse rather than being translated into practice (Dominelli, 2007). At a practical level, the process of engagement and relationship building with people is fundamental to good practice in this area. Plumb (2005) suggests that the main effects of abuse and oppression are damaged boundaries and powerlessness, and that this needs to be acknowledged in how services are offered. In particular, services need to be 'safe, accepting, empowering, nurturing, containing and appropriately structured. Negotiation rather than coercion is essential. They also need to offer unconditional acceptance, while retaining boundaries' (Plumb, 2005: 124). Social workers may also be key players in the initial assessment of emotional or psychological difficulties associated with trauma, abuse or disaster, and this can only be facilitated if initial relationships are experienced as accepting and positive, with particular attention being paid to issues of culture and language difference when working with people who have experience of fleeing from torture or civil unrest.

Signposting or referring to specialist agencies requires social work practitioners to be knowledgeable about what resources and services might be appropriate and available. It may be necessary to advocate for funding or other support, such as transport or child care to ensure that access is possible.

Looking After Yourself

As has already been suggested, it is important to be aware of your own needs for support as a social worker when working in highly charged and distressing situations. Harper (1993), describing the challenges of offering a support service after the Hillsborough disaster in 1989, when ninety-six people were crushed to death and many more were injured at a football stadium in Sheffield, refers to three areas of difficulty affecting workers. First was the presence of concurrent issues of loss in the workers' own lives; second was the impact of past memories, sometimes from childhood; and third was an upsurge in their work at key times or events relating to the disaster, such as the first Christmas or the inquest. Harper's experience confirms the importance of recognizing the need for staff support in order to prevent burn-out and to challenge any suggestion that workers are immune from the stress and pressures associated with responding to distress in people's lives, whether at the level of events affecting individuals, families or communities.

Activity

List some of the factors that may either promote or hinder creating a safe environment for working with people who have experienced trauma.

As a social worker, what can you do to help create safety within your own practice and service?

What potential sources of support can you identify for yourself when working in stressful situations?

Concluding Comments

This chapter has identified a number of areas where social workers need to be alert to a range of mental health difficulties including depression and anxiety, dual diagnosis and personality disorder. The importance of core social work skills, knowledge and values has been emphasized in working with individuals and their families and in contributing to providing interventions that are sensitive to issues of gender and culture. The current emphasis on CBT has also been acknowledged and a brief introduction to the therapy has been offered. Additionally, the potential contribution of social work in responding to trauma and disaster has been considered.

Further Reading

Foster, J. L. H. (2007) *Journeys through Mental Illness: Clients' Experiences and Understandings of Mental Distress*. Basingstoke: Palgrave Macmillan

Grant, A., Townend, M., Mulhern R. & Short, N. (2010) *Cognitive Behavioural Therapy in Mental Health Care*. 2nd edn. London: Sage

Greenberger, D. & Padesky, C. A. (1995) *Mind Over Mood: Change How You Feel By Changing the Way You Think*. New York: Guilford Press

Resources

Personality Disorder Programme: www.personalitydisorder.org.uk

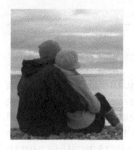

10 Working with People Experiencing Psychosis

Key points
• Working with a stress vulnerability model of psychosis
• The importance of engagement when working with people experiencing psychosis
• A collaborative approach to assessment, planning and intervention
• Promoting social work within the multiprofessional context

Introduction

This chapter will consider ways of working with people with psychosis, including schizophrenia or bipolar disorder, which can have a severe impact on the quality of life. It is relevant to note that whilst such difficulties may be designated as 'long-term', in reality the condition may be episodic, offering opportunities to support individuals in making choices and decisions about the support they require and to promote recovery.

A key theme is the importance of engagement and building relationships, emphasizing strengths and recovery-based approaches. Three 'Practice examples', based on the case studies of Stuart, Manjeet and Sharon, will be introduced and used to illustrate the application of the concepts in practice, including the importance of working with families.

As already discussed in Chapter 2, the dominance of the medical model of mental illness is open to challenge and critique from various perspectives and there are a number of conceptual and linguistic difficulties in defining what is meant by mental health and illness. Essentially, however, good practice for social workers and other like-minded practitioners relies on the application of shared models of understanding, including a social perspective, which can incorporate notions of recovery and social inclusion.

The chapter will begin by considering the fit between core social work values and approaches and the prevailing ethos of mental health service delivery in terms of recovery and the Ten Essential Shared Capabilities (National Institute for Mental Health in England/Sainsbury Centre for Mental Health Joint Workforce Support Unit, 2004; Care Sector Improvement Partnership/Royal College of Psychiatrists/Social Care Institute for Excellence, 2007). These will be developed further in relation to a case management model and a range of interventions.

Values and Approaches

The increasing attention being paid to recovery and social inclusion within the mental health agenda has been experienced as unsettling by some social workers, as social work values are recast as core to all aspects of mental health practice. Listening to the voices of service users, and working to challenge inequality and discrimination and to promote human rights and social justice, are intrinsic to social work, as are the language and practice of anti-oppressive practice and empowerment. However, this does present an important opportunity for social workers to demonstrate these values in practice and to work with colleagues to develop new and innovative ways of working that truly reflect this philosophy.

The introduction of the Ten Essential Shared Capabilities for the mental health workforce (National Institute for Mental Health in England/Sainsbury Centre for Mental Health Joint Workforce Support Unit, 2004), as set out in Figure 10.1, articulates this value base, providing an integrated framework which is intended to be shared and 'owned' within teams.

Reflection point

Consider each of the Ten Essential Shared Capabilities and how these might be translated into practice.

Do any of the points pose particular challenges in their implementation?

To what extent do they mirror social work values, and can you identify any differences or tensions between this framework and your own understanding of social work values?

Talk with a mental health professional who is not a social worker about their understanding of the Ten Essential Shared Capabilities and the 'fit' with their own professional value base.

Working in partnership

Respecting diversity

Practising ethically

Challenging inequality

Promoting recovery

Identifying people's needs and strengths

Providing service user-centred care

Making a difference

Promoting safety and positive risk taking

Personal development and learning

Figure 10.1   The Ten Essential Shared Capabilities
Source: National Institute for Mental Health in England/Sainsbury Centre for Mental Health Joint Workforce Support Unit (2004)

A major issue in developing interprofessional practice in mental health and in other areas of practice is the need to develop shared understanding and language to promote effective communication. This is a dynamic and sometimes difficult process but one which can result in greater understanding and increased potential for successful collaborative working.

Practice example

Jhoti is a newly qualified social worker based in a community mental health team. She has experience of working with occupational therapists in the past and whilst finding their contribution helpful from a practical perspective – for example, when working with someone being discharged from hospital – has not viewed occupational therapy as a profession working to challenge inequality. When she spends a day with Steve, an occupational therapy student, she is surprised to hear him refer to 'occupational justice' when discussing access to community-based facilities for people with long-term mental health difficulties. Further shared exploration of this term enables them both to realize that they share an approach to practice based on justice and challenging inequality and discrimination. Following this, Jhoti realizes that there may be more opportunities for shared working with occupational therapy colleagues than she had previously appreciated.

Working with other professionals requires a willingness to listen and learn from others and an openness to different ideas and thinking. These can be seen to contribute to the development of 'communities of practice' (Wenger, 1998), in which members can share vision and goals, repertoires of practice and language. At the same time there is a need to maintain confidence in your own professional contribution and to be able to tolerate uncertainty in exploring different approaches.

Frameworks for Practice

The term 'case management' was introduced in the UK (Audit Commission, 1986) to describe the co-ordination of care in the community for people with severe mental health difficulties. Initially there was some confusion between the different systems of 'case' and 'care' management being used by health and social workers respectively, with different understandings of case management. For some this involved a 'brokerage model' in which the role of the worker was to assess and co-ordinate services rather than deliver care themselves, while others espoused a view of case management more closely akin to the traditional social work model, in which the ongoing relationship between worker and service user was central.

The main framework for care for people requiring access to a range of services or deemed to be at a high level of risk is provided by the Care Programme Approach (CPA) (Department of Health, 2008b). This includes assessment and planning to meet a range of needs including psychiatric, psychological and social functioning, as well as crisis planning, risk, family, housing, financial, employment, education and physical health needs. Issues of equality, diversity and social inclusion should also be addressed. The Care Co-ordinator has the responsibility for ensuring that all aspects of care are co-ordinated, delivered and reviewed across all the agencies and systems involved and that continuity is maintained in the event that someone moves in and out of hospital or prison.

Within this overarching approach, the examples in this chapter will also refer to Bailey's five-stage approach (2002), introduced in Chapter 8, and draw on other frameworks for intervention such as Onyett's 'On-going Cycle of Work' (2003: 142). This has been modified below and each of the following phases will be considered in turn:

- engagement and relationship building;
- assessment;
- collaborative formulation;
- interventions to promote social inclusion;
- interventions to support wellbeing and recovery, including family work and relapse prevention;
- evaluation.

The collaborative development of a 'formulation' provides a rationale, explicitly shared between the service user and the worker, for making sense of the assessment and the accompanying interventions, based on a stress vulnerability model.

Social Work and Psychosocial Interventions

Psychosocial interventions (PSI) for people experiencing psychosis were introduced as a new approach to understanding and responding to the diagnosis of schizophrenia. Many nurses, occupational therapists and psychologists, along with doctors, social workers and support workers, have undertaken PSI training, contributing to the development of shared language and practice, supported by a growing evidence base for a range of interventions.

Stress vulnerability
a way of understanding the development of psychosis as a response to the interaction of psychological and environmental stressors with underlying vulnerability, including early life experiences, cognitive processing and genetic predisposition.

The introduction of PSI has had a mixed response from social work. On the one hand, this has been seen as other professions adopting a repertoire of approaches not unfamiliar to social work. On the other, the clinical discourse, use of validated assessment schedules and the introduction of a cognitive behavioural model do not necessarily fit comfortably with a social work approach. In order to ensure that PSI practice continues to develop, further critical appraisal of the complex professional discourses and dynamics involved may be required.

A detailed introduction to PSI is not possible in this text. However, some key concepts will be introduced, beginning with a **stress vulnerability** model of psychosis.

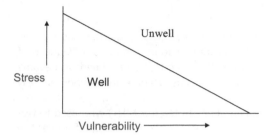

Figure 10.2   Stress vulnerability model
Source: Adapted from Zubin and Spring (1977: 110)

Understanding psychosis using a stress vulnerability model

Within the stress vulnerability model, the concept of vulnerability is seen as 'a process that increases the liability for mental disorder but of itself is insufficient to cause disorder' (Goldberg & Goodyer, 2005: 168). This is considered to include: genetics, cognitive processing, developmental processes, early life experience and personality traits, although the order in which these occur and their relative influences and interactions are unknown.

The overall stressors associated with the model include critically, emotionally involved attitudes towards the person, an overstimulating social environment and stressful life events. Figure 10.2 is based on the work of Zubin and Spring (1977) and demonstrates how increased vulnerability, shown towards the right of the horizontal axis, lowers the level of stress required to become unwell.

The interaction of vulnerability and stressors is unique for each person, and this of itself offers a valuable counter to notions of 'them and us' in that any one of us may, given sufficient stress, experience aspects of psychosis. Furthermore, the model offers twin opportunities both to reduce stressors and to develop coping strategies.

Engagement

Building relationships is an essential first stage of the process of working with a service user, many of whom have experienced rejection and discrimination in other parts of their lives. For some, previous experiences of seeking help have also been distressing and negative.

The 'Practice example' concerns a social worker in an Adult Social Care Team, Hari, and his first contact with Stuart, a 48-year-old man.

Practice example

Hari has been asked to visit Stuart, who lives with his mother. Stuart's mother has recently been diagnosed with cancer and is becoming unable to care for Stuart, who had a diagnosis of schizophrenia twenty-five years ago. There is a concern in the team that Stuart needs to become less dependent on his mother and that over the years he has become increasingly socially isolated.

Hari contacts a nurse from the local community mental health team (CMHT) who used to visit Stuart to monitor his medication. She confirms that Stuart has not been in hospital for over five years but that previously he had several admissions under the Mental Health Act, which had caused him and his mother considerable distress. Hari decides to arrange a joint visit with a colleague who is already involved in undertaking an assessment of Stuart's mother.

When Hari and his colleague arrive Stuart quickly leaves the room, and Hari observes him going into the well-kept garden outside. After a few minutes Hari follows him and asks if he can join him. Stuart is very wary but responds briefly and quietly to Hari's positive comments about the garden. Stuart appears to be unconfident and unpractised in conversation but agrees that Hari can visit again. Before he goes Hari asks Stuart if he is worried about his mother, and Stuart nods. Hari suggests that maybe they could talk about that a bit more on his next visit.

In many respects this may not seem like a piece of dynamic social work practice, and to many hard-pressed social workers with busy caseloads the seemingly slow progress that might be involved may seem a luxury. However, Hari is clearly demonstrating key social work competences in the skilful way in which he is beginning to build a relationship with Stuart, drawing on the information he has gathered and making good use of various observational and non-verbal cues when he visits Stuart. There is a purposeful nature to this seemingly informal approach, which paves the way for further contact with a vulnerable and isolated man whose previous contact with services may have, on occasions, been upsetting and frightening. By allowing time to build trust and demonstrate respect, Hari is able to begin to build a more rounded picture of Stuart that will inform his assessment, in keeping with Bailey's first stage of practice (see Figure 8.2).

Other key elements of engagement may also be present in this example, including the beginnings of an empathic response to Stuart's situation with respect to his mother's illness. A particular feature of engagement is frequently the capacity of the worker to demonstrate the practical advantages that may be involved. Whilst these may not be present so far in this example, for many people attention to the detail and challenges of everyday life – the broken washing machine or worries about paying the rent – is valued at a practical level and demonstrates concern and interest (Wilson, 2002).

Assessment

A strengths approach to assessment

A strengths model, now widely used in mental health practice, was initially developed within social work (Rapp & Wintersteen, 1989; Saleebey, 1997), and continues to offer a relevant approach to practice. In particular the value of a strengths approach has been its 'fit' with a recovery-based approach, as will be seen in the discussion that follows.

Once an initial relationship has been established it is important to remain focused on the reason for contact and to consider how the worker can support the service user in identifying and moving towards their goals. In the 'Practice example' above, the initial referral may have been to find alternative accommodation for Stuart, whereas he may prefer to stay in the house where he has been living for many years. He may also want to prioritize making friends or learning new skills. Whilst it might initially appear that Stuart has some challenges to face, it is important that he is supported in making decisions about his future.

Focusing on strengths rather than deficits draws attention to what Stuart wants for the future and the resources he already has that may help him to achieve these. A strengths model also asks about hopes and dreams, and whilst these may not always be achievable, a discussion of these can open up new ideas and possibilities as well as providing a powerful motivational drive towards change.

Figure 10.3 offers a number of questions about discovering strengths and provides an alternative to some of the frequently asked questions about problems. An important component of questions such as these is that they can convey hope for the future. Without hope any one of us can feel that life is pointless, yet all too often workers as well as service users have little hope that things could change for the better.

Reflection point

Read through the lists of questions and reflect on your response to them. Are there any which might feel were difficult to ask? Do you think that there are some situations where it might feel hard or uncomfortable to ask them? If so, what is it about the questions – or the potential answers – that makes you respond in this way?

When considering hope, workers can often become concerned that they are raising hope inappropriately or creating expectations which may be unrealistic. How can you respond if someone wants to recapture lost relationships or buy a house in Spain? In reality most service users are all too well aware of the limitations they may encounter in pursuing their dreams. However, it is possible to harness the desires

Discovering strengths

Survival questions:

How have you managed to get through/survive/thrive given the challenges you have encountered?

What have you learned about yourself as you faced these challenges?

Which of these difficulties have given you special strength/insight/skill?

Support questions:

Who has given you understanding, support and/or guidance?

Who are the people you have been able to depend upon?

How did you find them – or how did they find you?

Exception questions:

When things were going well, what was different?

What parts of your experience would you like to relive or recapture?

Possibility questions:

What do you want out of life now?

What are your hopes/dreams/aspirations?

What/Who is helping you move towards these?

How can I help you achieve your goals?

Esteem questions:

When people say good things about you, what are they likely to say?

What is it about your life that you feel proud about?

When was it you began to believe that you might achieve some of the things you wanted in life?

What do you enjoy in life?

Figure 10.3   The strengths approach
Source: Adapted from Saleebey (1997)

and feelings wrapped up with some dreams and build on these to create positive changes. In some cases discussion of what would be entailed realistically to achieve a seemingly unobtainable goal may create other possible avenues to explore.

The 'Practice example' introduces Manjeet, a young woman whose aspirations were initially dashed by her experiences of bipolar disorder, but for whom the application of a strengths approach by her social worker begins to offer hope for the future.

Practice example

Manjeet is 26 and has had several episodes of mania, one of which was followed by a period of depression. She has also experienced delusional beliefs. A lengthy period in hospital led to her giving up her university course in biological sciences, which she had hoped would enable her to become a vet.

Marie, her social worker, decides to work from a strengths perspective and asks her about her hopes and dreams for the future. In exploring these with Manjeet, Marie listens carefully and respects her ideas, suggesting that they consider how these might be achieved. Together they identify a number of activities that would help Manjeet begin to move towards her goals, including attending a part-time return-to-study module at the local college, where there is an excellent student support service that will help Manjeet in re-establishing herself as a student. Additionally, Manjeet is interested in undertaking some voluntary work with animals, and Marie is able to provide information about various opportunities that would provide this.

Manjeet's social worker also uses a strengths assessment (Figure 10.4), which she has found to be helpful in identifying positive resources and experiences that may be useful for Manjeet to draw on. A strengths assessment also provides a framework in which to consider all aspects of Manjeet's life rather than focusing solely on the experience of symptoms and pathology.

Other assessments

Time lines

As with a strengths approach, a collaborative approach to assessment underpins the drawing of a time line, which can assist in making sense of complex life events. Similarly, the use of time lines is a valuable tool in any aspect of social work assessment, being easily adapted and transferred to different situations.

Sharon has experienced mental health difficulties for a number of years, and a time line was found to be helpful in identifying some of the stressful events that she had experienced as well as some positive experiences. In the version in Figure 10.5, produced by Sharon with the support of her social worker, the left-hand and right-hand columns contain the positives and negatives respectively. Alternative representations of a chronological history could be produced with drawing or other more visual means of conveying information.

Structured assessment tools

In some circumstances additional assessments may be introduced to explore the specific details of individual experiences further. For example, the KGV assessment (Lancashire, 1998) offers a

	What has worked in the past?	What is happening at present?	What do I want in the future?
Name: Manjeet		*Date:* January 2011	
Daily living including housing	Lived at home in first year at university	Still living at home but feel as if I am being looked after by my parents	Would like to be more independent again
Financial	Had a small student loan and this meant I could spend my own money	Receiving benefits but contributing to household expenses and there is not much left over	Would like to have enough money to be able to go out more
Occupation/Education	Started at university to study biological sciences	Nothing	I want to go back to university and study to become a vet
Social and spiritual supports	Had friends at school but have now lost touch with them. No contact with anyone from university	See best friend, Sunita, once a week. Sister is very supportive. However, I feel quite isolated from other people my age	Would like to have the opportunity to meet more people and make some new friends
Health, including medication	Used to be very healthy	Often lacking in energy and tired due to medication	I want more energy
Recreation/Leisure	Was involved in lots of school activities	Bored and frustrated at home	Something but not sure what

Figure 10.4   Manjeet's strengths assessment

Phenomenological emphasizes first-hand, subjective experience and is concerned with interpretation and meaning rather than notions of absolute truth.

phenomenological approach to building up a detailed picture of experiences including unusual thoughts and beliefs, hallucinations or voices, depression and suicidality, based on the experience of the individual concerned and through the use of prompt questions to ascertain frequency, duration and intensity of each indicator. Whilst specific training is required in order for this assessment to be used as an outcome measure or research tool, the collaborative use of detailed questions can be used to identify positive coping strategies as well as negative experiences. The KGV may also be followed up with the use of specific assessments to explore areas of shared concern further, such as hallucinations or delusions.

Born	1976	
Brother Alan born	1979	Mum unwell and in hospital for 5 months. Looked after by Auntie Maggie and her boyfriend – he smacked me for being naughty.
Started school	1980	Mum and Dad split up. and Dad moved away.
	1983	Mum not well again and I was sent to stay with Gran in Newcastle. Missed a lot of school. Alan stayed with Auntie Maggie.
Came home to live with mum and her new boyfriend, John	1984	Had to go to a new school. Got called names because my dad was black.
	1987	Changed schools and didn't have any friends.
Drama teacher picked me for the school play	1990	Mum has another baby, Ellen, but I had to babysit and look after her a lot. No time for homework and seeing friends.
Enjoying drama at school and asked to join a drama group	1991	Mum still not well so had to look after Ellen and Alan. Missed more school so couldn't do drama.
Left school	1992	Wanted to go to college and do drama but poor exam results.
Met boyfriend – Martin	1993	
Go to live with Martin in his bedsit	1994	Feel very down and get lonely as Martin went out with his friends every night.
	1995	Gran dies. Mum in hospital and I had to go home to help with Ellen. Used to think that people were talking about me when I went out.
Got my own flat	1996	Split up with Martin.
Got a job as a waitress and met new boyfriend	1997	Flat broken into while I was in bed.
	1997	Took an overdose after new relationship broke up.
	1998	Alan comes to stay but his friends were always visiting. One of them attacked me one night. Went to the police but they didn't do anything.
	2000	Voices in my head started. Sometimes they were OK but often they said I was evil. Thought it was the neighbours.
	2001	Went into hospital for 6 weeks after getting into a fight in the street.
Moved into new flat to get away from the neighbours. Met Annette, who lived next door – went out sometimes	2002	Couldn't get work – my medication affected me badly. Spent most of my time on my own in the flat. Mum not well and called me a lot to try and get me to go and help her. Often borrowed money.
	2004	Voices still bad and told me to kill myself. Took another overdose. Ended up in hospital again. Given a diagnosis of schizophrenia.
New boyfriend – Joss	2005	Became pregnant but lost the baby – the doctor said I wouldn't have been a fit mother anyway because of my illness.
	2006	Very depressed and sent back into hospital for 5 months. Split up with Joss. Alan went to stay in the flat and things got trashed.
Get back together with Joss and moved in with him. He helped me to cope when Mum was in hospital	2007	
	2009	Mum died of cancer. Voices bad again.

Figure 10.5 Sharon's time line

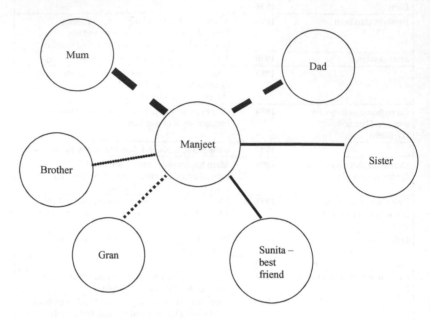

Figure 10.6   Manjeet's ecogram

Ecograms and social network maps

Ecograms are used in many areas of social work and are relevant in mental health work when considering the important relationships and networks that affect people's lives. Figure 10.6 contains an example from Marie's work with Manjeet.

As they draw out the ecomap, Manjeet talks about her relationships and depicts them with dotted lines to show that there is currently not a lot of connection, dashed lines to show conflict and solid lines to indicate a strong and positive connection. Her social worker recognizes that this information is valuable and will help inform her work with Manjeet, and maybe later on with her family. The social worker is also concerned that she recognizes the cultural issues that may be relevant and notes that that this might be an important issue to consider further.

Social network maps are also used within a PSI approach, building on the evidence that intense and stressful family relationships may increase the risk of relapse (Kavanagh, 1992). The use of a social network map to identify relationships creates opportunities for these to be reviewed and interventions offered to reduce stress and increase positive contact.

Collaborative Formulation: Weighing Up the Options

A stress vulnerability formulation is a way of bringing together the information gathered as part of the assessment process and using it to make sense of the individual's current situation. In essence it offers a rationale to help make sense of the person's mental health experiences, forming a story that provides the basis for taking the work forward.

A user-friendly version of the model has been illustrated as a bucket (Brabban & Turkington, 2002). This can be easily drawn and discussed, with the bucket representing the resources and/or vulnerability of the person to manage stress. Unlike most buckets in everyday life, this bucket requires holes for drainage, which can be explained as the coping mechanisms that may be available to the individual. However, these can be become blocked, for example by the use of alcohol or street drugs, or unblocked through the development of new coping strategies or other interventions including medication. Liquid dripping into the bucket represents the various stressors that the person may be experiencing. If these come to exceed the capacity of the bucket, and in the absence of other ways of managing them, the bucket will overflow. This is seen as representing the experience of becoming unwell. Whilst the metaphor of the bucket may not work for everyone, there is considerable value in using everyday language to make sense of experience, as a possible formulation for Sharon below demonstrates:

> *Formulation for Sharon:*
>
> Life was difficult as a child as your mum was not able to look after you due to her health problems and you were cared for by different people who did not always treat you well. Together with your experiences of racism at school, it was hard for you to feel positive about yourself as you were growing up and this continued into your adult life, making you more vulnerable to some of the stressful events that happened. These included losing your grandmother, your flat being broken into and the stress of caring for other family members. Your voices started at a time when you were at a particularly low point and have recurred at other difficult times.

The collaborative nature of developing the formulation cannot be overemphasized; nor can its dynamic quality, developing over time as new information and experience become available. The collaborative formulation is the basis for setting goals, providing a guide for further work, which, for Sharon, might include a range of interventions to promote recovery and improve her quality of life as well as helping her to manage her mental health.

Weighing up the options therefore requires considering the priorities for taking action. Working with a model of recovery means that this does not necessarily entail addressing 'symptoms' but can involve a range of alternative strategies that reflect the individual's own wishes and goals. At times these may create some dilemmas for social workers, who may experience some tensions not only between the service user's wishes and their own, but also with the priorities of their team or organization.

Reflection point

As you read this chapter, think about some of the dilemmas that might arise in working with Sharon, Manjeet or Stuart in terms of conflicting priorities.
   How might you try to manage these?

Interventions to Promote Social Inclusion

Moving on to consider interventions, it is important to recognize that the use of holistic and user-focused assessments such as have been described here could also be seen as interventions with their own intrinsic value. This may lie in the personal narrative or story-telling that emerges, increased self-respect and dignity associated with being invited to participate within a spirit of collaborative inquiry and the recognition of individual decisions and choices.

It is also important that interventions are embedded firmly within a care plan associated with the CPA, ensuring that all those involved are clear about the various contributions that they may be making to the work. For example, as Hari's work with Stuart develops, Hari may involve a mental health support worker to assist Stuart in joining a local gardening group. A nurse colleague may help to reassess Stuart's medication and monitor side effects. Links with other agencies and organizations are also likely to feature, as working towards social inclusion will necessarily involve organizations outside of health and social services.

Personalization

Personalization is central to care planning and is likely to develop further with the increasing use of direct payments and individual budgets. This will create new opportunities for social workers to act as advocates, navigators, brokers, advisers, risk assessors and auditors, as well as providing specific services themselves. It is also anticipated that social workers will find themselves involved in the design of new care provision, drawing on knowledge and skills in community working and development (Carr, 2008). Whilst these issues of policy are discussed in more detail in Chapter 3, the implications for practice are significant. For example, whilst initial discussions might have suggested that Stuart would be unable to live independently once his mother was no longer able to care for him, the availability of direct payments and a personalized budget could purchase a range of tailored services that will enable him to stay in his own home.

Social networks

Repper and Perkins (2003) remind us that mental health services have often focused on symptoms rather than the other important aspects of people's lives, and that by the time attention is turned to 'rehabilitation', opportunities and hope have been damaged. Repper and Perkins emphasize the need to address this in three interrelated ways:

- hope-inspiring relationships;
- facilitating personal adaptation – coping strategies and skills;
- promoting social access and inclusion.

Whilst greater attention is now being paid to maintaining and strengthening contact with families and friends by all mental health practitioners, social workers have particular expertise and experience in this area. Contacts provided by family and friends also help provide links to other resources such as voluntary activities, paid employment and wider social networks.

Reflection point

Think back to the activity at the end of Chapter 5 and the list of community facilities that you may have identified. Consider how these might be relevant to the needs of Stuart, Sharon or Manjeet. What other resources might be available that you could investigate as ways of increasing social networking opportunities and promoting social inclusion?

Identifying opportunities and resources is only the first step, as it may not be enough simply to provide the information, especially if the particular service user is unconfident and has previously experienced discouragement. A strengths approach can be helpful in identifying current and past activities, and assist in recalling effective strategies that have worked before. The worker's own spirit of optimism and hope will also help build confidence in picking up old interests or tackling new activities.

Practice example

Sharon's time line shows that she has survived a number of difficulties in her life: it may take some time to rebuild her confidence and for her to have hope for the future. Her social worker suggests a number of ways in which they could work together to increase her involvement in community-based activities and networks gradually, and Sharon agrees that this is worth a try. Sharon's interest and ability in drama might be a good place to start, but together they decide that this might be too big a step at this stage. However, they agree to keep this in mind as a goal for the future whilst initially concentrating on building Sharon's confidence. The social worker has previously had some contact with a local voluntary sector mental health organization that runs a women's group, and she wonders whether Sharon might be interested in this. With Sharon's cautious agreement they arrange a meeting with the group worker. The group is small and offers a supportive environment which will help to build Sharon's confidence and also offer some social contact.

Working to increase social networks can be seen as involving two main areas of activity. This involves first being familiar with community resources and building up your own network of contacts, and then working with the individual to support them in this part of their journey to recovery. Repper and Perkins (2003) address these issues in some detail, and a summary of various aspects of both these activities is outlined in Figure 10.7.

Employment and education

For Manjeet's social worker, issues regarding education and employment emerged early on in their discussions about strengths and hopes for the future. Together they were able to plan out how Manjeet could gradually increase her activities and work up to returning to education. An important aspect of this plan was to ensure that a range of supports

---

In the community

Gaining information and building up a resources bank that can also be shared with other
    colleagues

Making personal contact with services and organizations in order to build trust

Providing general information about mental health and the importance of social networks

Keeping in touch with the agencies concerned and providing a safety net or point of contact if
    any issues arise; offering advice and support in handling sensitive situations

With individuals

Plan small steps but be clear about where they are leading

Identify possible difficulties and strategies to overcome them

Be prepared to 'go the extra mile' on occasions, including joining in new activities and acting
    as a role model in learning new things

Build in other sources of support and encouragement

Celebrate success

Figure 10.7   Increasing social networks
Source: Adapted from Repper and Perkins (2003)

was in place as Manjeet's parents were anxious that she did not over-stretch herself and should maybe give up her career plans.

Interventions to Support Wellbeing and Recovery

In addition to the approaches described above, which have the express purpose of increasing social inclusion, there may also be a need to address particular issues that may otherwise act as obstacles to overall wellbeing and recovery. Three different areas will be considered here, and again relevant points will be illustrated by continuing the stories of Sharon and Manjeet.

Relapse prevention

Work to reduce the risk of relapse is often a key feature of early interventions when psychosis is first experienced, and may also be useful in long-standing situations. The purpose is to identify some of the early indicators that someone is becoming unwell in order for interventions to be offered before things deteriorate further. With hindsight, individuals and those close to them can often recall early changes in their behaviour that took place before they were seen to be unwell, and this has been called the **prodromal phase**. When some of these changes have been identified, a relapse prevention plan is drawn up to enable assistance to be sought and offered at an early stage if and when any future difficulties recur. As with all of the interventions being discussed here, a collaborative approach to this work is essential.

Prodromal phase
changes in an individual's behaviour, thoughts and mood in the period before relapse occurs.

Cognitive behavioural therapy

The notion that symptoms of psychosis such as delusions and hallucinations are, first, irrational and unrelated to reality and, second, not amenable to interventions has been challenged by the work of Marius Romme and others (Romme & Escher, 1993; Baker, 1995; Coleman & Smith, 1997), drawing attention to the number of people in the general population who have heard voices in the absence of any other indicators of mental health difficulties. Rather than necessarily being seen as a symptom of illness, the 'normalizing' of hearing voices offers an alternative to the prejudice and stigma that many people have encountered, offering new ways of understanding this experience and potential for spiritual, creative and other holistic interpretations. For some people, the voices may be comforting or a positive presence in their lives, whilst for others, strategies to manage the voices may help to reduce the level of intrusion or impact they have on everyday life.

There is also evidence regarding the success of cognitive behavioural approaches to managing unusual beliefs or delusions, similarly recognizing that they are dynamic, often related to experience, and may vary over time and place in relation to the strength of conviction with which they are held, their duration, frequency, intensity and the level of distress which may be experienced. This is endorsed by guidance from the National Institute for Health and Clinical Excellence (2009c), which recommends that anyone with a diagnosis of schizophrenia should be offered sixteen planned, one-to-one sessions of cognitive behavioural therapy (CBT) from an early stage of treatment. Similar recommendations also exist for family work, which is discussed further below.

It is important to note that the following discussion is offered so that social workers are aware of the potential of such interventions, and is not intended to be a 'how to' guide for working with unusual beliefs. The interested reader is recommended to explore this further with additional reading, training and supervision to support their own professional development in this area.

A basic model of CBT has already been introduced in Chapter 9. Here we shall consider how Sharon's social worker, Denise, discusses the possible benefits of this approach with a colleague trained as a cognitive behavioural therapist. Denise learns that working with unusual beliefs would begin by considering less strongly held beliefs that may cause some distress for the person rather than those held with a high degree of conviction. Her colleague explains that the person is not asked to change their belief and adopt a new one but simply to consider the evidence for that belief. It is the evidence rather than the belief that is challenged, and the individual would be asked to think first about any possible alternatives to this evidence – a 'verbal re-attribution' – before working with the therapist to undertake a behavioural 'experiment' or 'reattribution' to test this out.

Previously Denise had felt unsure about the value of CBT, but this discussion leads her to thinks that it might be helpful for Sharon at some point in the future, especially regarding her belief that the neighbours are talking about her. Denise can imagine that within a trusting and collaborative working relationship, Sharon might be able to look at some other ways of making sense of this experience and possibly test out some of the alternative explanations. Whilst this might not completely remove the belief, it might lessen its impact and potentially help Sharon to feel safer at home.

Family work

The families of someone affected by psychosis can make a vital contribution to recovery, although they may need support to tackle the various challenges that may arise. As we have already seen in Chapter 1, families have sometimes been viewed negatively, not recognized for their positive contribution and often left perplexed and distressed by what is happening.

Working with families to provide education and to maximize effective coping strategies is now recognized as an important component of the range of interventions offered to people with a diagnosis of schizophrenia or bipolar disorder (National Institute for Health and Clinical Excellence, 2006, 2009c). However, the reality is that family work is not widely implemented or available because of service constraints. It is also important to note that family work means working with whoever is significant to the individual and is not restricted to the conventional family unit: in some situations, residential care teams might also be considered to be an appropriate focus for such work.

In continuing our discussion of Marie's work with Manjeet, the possibility of family work is explored further in line with the suggestion that communication training and problem-solving skills are appropriate interventions in families where someone has a diagnosis of bipolar disorder (National Institute for Health and Clinical Excellence, 2006; Goodwin, 2009).

Practice example

Marie is aware that there are some tensions between Manjeet and her family and that so far these have not been addressed, partly because Manjeet is keen to strengthen and maintain her sense of herself as an independent adult. The social worker is also aware that whilst she has established a good working relationship with Manjeet, working with Manjeet's Sikh family from a different cultural background may also present its own challenges. However, over a period of months it appears that the situation at home has been becoming more difficult and is threatening to undermine Manjeet's efforts to go back to college. Manjeet reports that there are frequent arguments about how much time she is spending in her bedroom and how this is viewed by her parents as a symptom of her illness.

Marie discusses the situation with another social work colleague who has considerable experience of family work, and who offers to co-work with Marie. An initial meeting with Manjeet, her parents and siblings provides an opportunity for introductions and some general discussion about what the work would entail. Manjeet does not find this easy but is surprised at some of the positive statements made by her brother and sister. A second meeting is arranged and it is agreed that this will focus on the different ways in which the family members make sense of Manjeet's 'illness' and will provide a space for Manjeet to describe the work she has been doing with Marie, being careful to ensure that Manjeet is in control of the information that she feels comfortable in sharing with her parents and siblings. This is successful in allowing Manjeet's voice to be heard within the family, who are able to see that this offers an understandable rationale for Manjeet's difficulties. It also offers an alternative to her parents' view that she is suffering from an incurable illness and needs to be treated as an invalid. However, tensions about how much time Manjeet is spending time in her room remain unresolved and a third session is planned to introduce a six-step problem-solving approach.

This third session involves everyone in thinking about the 'problem' of Manjeet staying in her room and how this could be described in a neutral fashion. It is eventually described as *'The family don't feel they see enough of Manjeet in the evenings at home.'* Linked to this is a goal for *'The family to spend more quality time together.'*

A range of possible solutions is proposed, including cooking a meal together or watching TV, going out together or visiting Manjeet's sister, who lives nearby, so that Manjeet couldn't escape to her room. These are then considered in terms of their respective advantages and disadvantages, and increasingly everyone seems to became more relaxed, recognizing that it is fine for someone to spend some time alone and that this is to be expected in a family. The final solution is that the family will spend time together on two prearranged evenings a week and that this will involve preparing and eating a shared meal or watching a TV programme that they will all enjoy. Manjeet's brother is charged with making sure that Manjeet's parents do not interfere with Manjeet spending time alone in her room on other evenings, and their older sister is to check in every week and ask about the plans.

A follow-up family session two weeks later finds that so far the plan is working and that the number of arguments has decreased.

Whilst it would be unrealistic to suggest that such positive outcomes are always easily achieved, this 'Practice example' demonstrates the importance of recognizing the strengths and support that can be available within families and the value of involving family members, where appropriate, when working with individuals.

Details of the six-step problem-solving strategy are contained within Figure 10.8. Although intended for working with families, many people have also found that the process can be valuable in resolving problems in other settings and contexts, both personal and professional.

Evaluation

Onyett's final phase is evaluation. It is important to allow time to reflect on the effectiveness of the work that has been undertaken and for a review of the interventions in collaboration with the individual and, where appropriate, their family. This is also in line with stages 4 and 5 of Bailey's model, referred to earlier in this chapter and introduced in Chapter 8. Rather than being an end point, this appraisal, in terms of both the work that has been carried out and the worker's own personal learning, should form the basis of further work and development,

---

1. What exactly is the problem or goal? Discuss until this is clear and specific.

2. List all possible solutions. Include everyone's ideas and suggestions, even the ridiculous.

3. Highlight the main advantages and disadvantages of each solution.

4. Choose the 'best' realistic solution.

5. Plan exactly how the solution will be carried out. Try to involve everyone in the plan.

   Consider what might go wrong and introduce ways of overcoming this.

6. Review progress

Figure 10.8   Six-step problem-solving strategy
Source: Adapted from Falloon and Graham-Hole (1994) and from Gamble and Brennan (2000: 189)

beginning the cycle again. This may mean negotiating or renegotiating goals to reflect changing circumstances, and adjusting care plans and interventions in response to these.

The Team and Organizational Context for Mental Health Social Work

It will be clear from this chapter that social workers working with people experiencing mental health difficulties may be based in a range of settings, including adult social care teams in the local authority social service department and multidisciplinary mental health teams. In some areas there may be integrated NHS Care Trust arrangements. Some of the examples given concern the social worker based in a community mental health team, and this may mean that the social worker is employed by the local authority, which also provides professional social work management and supervision, but on a day-to-day basis is effectively a member of a multidisciplinary team, whose other members may be employed by the NHS. Increasingly, other services and agencies are also involved in the provision of mental health services, including the private, charitable and voluntary sectors, and such arrangements may be made on the basis of commissioning and tendering of services, sometimes involving collaborative partnerships. The spectrum of health care may also include home treatment and crisis intervention teams, early interventions, assertive outreach teams, inpatient beds and day treatment services.

Opportunities for social work are likely to exist in these and other new, innovative developments as they arise, each offering its own professional and organizational challenges as the complex mosaic of services continues to evolve. Increasing service user and carer involvement and the introduction of the personalization agenda, whilst being welcomed, also require new thinking and approaches to practice. This can require a continuing process of dialogue and negotiation with other colleagues and a level of confidence in articulating the distinctive role and contribution of social work.

Activity

Find out about the mental health teams and services in your area and map these out, identifying the various health and social care organizations involved.

To what extent are these co-ordinated and coterminous within one geographical area, or do they cross other boundaries of local and health authorities?

Consider how easy or difficult it might be for a service user or their family to find out about services and how to access them.

Concluding Comments

One of the continuing challenges for social workers in mental health settings, particularly in multidisciplinary teams, is to manage the delicate balance between the unique and specific contribution of the social work role and the shared sense of mental health practice, held in common with other team members and exemplified in notions of core mental health competences and the Ten Essential Shared Capabilities. This chapter has attempted to offer an integrated approach to working with people with long-term mental health difficulties, drawing on fundamental social work knowledge and values whilst integrating some of the knowledge and interventions drawn from the current practices of a range of mental health professionals.

Further Reading

Harris, N., Williams, S. & Bradshaw, T. (eds) (2002) *Psychosocial Interventions for People with Schizophrenia*. Basingstoke: Palgrave Macmillan

Repper, J. & Perkins, R. (2003) *Social Inclusion and Recovery: A Model for Mental Health Practice*. London: Bailliere Tindall

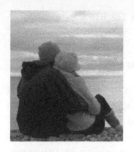

11 Interprofessional Working in Response to Risk

Key points

- The contested nature of risk discourse
- Integrating assessment and management of risk and dangerousness
- Recognition of risk for service users, including neglect, exclusion, self-harm and suicide
- Involving service users in risk assessment and management, including responding to crises/advance directives
- Legislative and statutory functions, including the role of the Approved Mental Health Professional
- Specific areas of practice, including forensic social work and mental health and child protection
- The contribution of social work to integrated services and the 'joined-up' agenda

Introduction

The imperative for 'joined-up working' lies at the heart of current health and social care policy and continues to be emphasized as a consistent theme in any inquiry involving issues of risk or where events have ended in tragedy. This chapter will begin by examining the ways in which risk is socially constructed and how this influences both policy and professional practice. The contribution and role of social workers in the multidisciplinary team will then be explored, emphasizing the importance of interprofessional working in the assessment and management of situations involving issues of risk and dangerousness from a range of different practice areas, including forensic mental health and child protection. Positive ways of working in response to some of the challenges and tensions will be identified, drawing on examples from real-life inquiries and the lessons for practice offered. Finally the chapter will return to the theme of interprofessional and multi-agency working, recognizing that this is not only key to improving practice in situations where issues of risk and dangerousness are seen to be involved, but also essential in promoting recovery and social inclusion for people experiencing mental health difficulties. This discussion will acknowledge the role that social work can play as part of the wider agenda for joined-up working.

Setting the Context of 'Risk' in Social Work

The concept of risk is rarely absent from discussions concerning mental health and illness and also features strongly in the wider realm of social work literature and theory. The title of this chapter itself suggests that risk is a key theme in social work and mental health practice and that this is shared with other professionals working in this area. Delving beyond official policy and practice guidance, however, leads to the recognition that the discourse of risk as frequently presented is contested and fraught with uncertainty.

A number of commentators have challenged the current preoccupation with risk both in society in general and more specifically in relation to social work practice. A critical sociological perspective (Giddens, 1991; Beck, 1992; Furedi, 1997), has drawn attention to the way in which risk avoidance is central to modernity. Increasing scientific knowledge, accompanied by technological developments, is viewed as having the potential to reduce the anxieties and uncertainties associated with living in contemporary society, such as climate change, conflict, economic crisis and disease. Suggestions that the 'risks' of a range of social, political and economic threats are increasing, in both the national and international arenas, are met, in turn, with increasing efforts to manage and reduce the likelihood of the threat. Within this paradigm the apparent consensus that risk is inevitably associated with danger, and must be avoided by any means, has created an array of organizational and bureaucratic procedures within a broader culture of blame when things do go wrong.

With regard to social work, Thompson associates the current preoccupation with risk with a shift from 'an emphasis on care and support for vulnerable and disadvantaged members of the community to a stronger focus on perceiving certain members of the community as a threat to wider society' (2010: 50). In doing so, he and others (Kemshall, 2002; Webb, 2006) raise important questions about the nature of social work and the extent to which issues of human rights and social justice, as set out in the definition considered in the Introduction to this text, can be seen as pivotal in an environment where there is increasing emphasis on managerial and organizational procedures intended to minimize risk. Examples of such practices can be seen in relation to child protection and the proliferation of monitoring and surveillance systems, one instance being increasing demands for criminal record checks. Paradoxically, there is increasing recognition that these are themselves inadequate and no guarantee of safety. Additionally, systems of risk and assessment bring their own dangers including the risk of inaccurate assessments, both false positives and false negatives, which carry their own potentially negative consequences. As is pointed out by a report on social work and risk assessment produced by the Scottish Executive (2007), there is increasing reliance on risk assessment tools being used to replace rather than inform professional judgement.

A critical stance on risk also raises a fundamental question as to whether the world has in fact become more dangerous or there is a greater preoccupation with risk and safety. In answering this question in relation to social work, O'Sullivan (2009) suggests that, rather than risk being understood as avoidable, it needs to be managed in a critical and creative fashion, recognizing the potential benefits as well as negative consequences of any particular course of action. Smith (2010) draws attention to the need for the social work profession to eschew claims to perfect knowledge which might be seen as ultimately eliminating high-profile child protection or other tragedies. Instead, principles of empowerment and self-determination, supported by collaborative working and the development of 'mutual problem solving strategies' (Smith 2010: 10), are proposed as key components of transformational and critical practice.

Reflection point

Drawing on your own life experience or from social work, identify examples of monitoring and surveillance which have been introduced in response to concerns about risk.
  Can you think of any negative as well as any positive implications of these examples?
  Are there any issues of human rights or social justice involved?

Risk, Dangerousness and Mental Health

To look more specifically at mental health and risk it is useful to begin by acknowledging the high level of concern and anxiety regarding mental illness, risk and danger in the media and public imagination. Annual surveys of attitudes to mental illness (TNS UK, 2009, 2010) suggest that there continues to be a significant level of suspicion regarding the risks to others posed by people with a mental illness, with approximately one third of respondents indicating that someone with a mental illness would be 'prone to violence', contributing to a long history of such stereotypical associations of mental illness with violence. (At the same time, however, a similar proportion agreed with the statement that 'Less emphasis should be placed on protecting the public from people with mental illness' (TNS UK, 2009: 3).) This theme was fuelled at the end of the twentieth century by what was seen as the 'failure' of community care, and public protection was a key driver for the modernization of mental health policy and legislation. The amendment of the 1983 legislation by the Mental Health Act 2007 (see Chapter 4) included what was widely viewed as the contentious provision for compulsory treatment in the community. Ramon (2005) points out that this preoccupation with mental health risk in Britain, whilst similar to those in North America and Australia, is not reflected in concerns elsewhere in Europe, where there is no comparable legislation for community treatment to address seemingly similar populations and levels of harm.

Events such as the killing of Isabel Schwarz, a social worker, by a former client in 1984 and of Jonathan Zito, a man unknown to the perpetrator, Christopher Clunis, in 1992 continue to be embedded within this debate, alongside more recent events. These include the murder in 2004 of Denis Finnegan by John Barrett (Finnegan was cycling through Richmond Park and Barrett was on leave from hospital) and of Tina Stevenson by Benjamin Holiday in 2005, discussed below (*Times Online*, 3 December 2006). In many of these and other similar cases, there are clear indicators that people were not well served or supported by mental health services, and that a failure of care contributed to the situation. It is impossible to believe that similar tragedies will not occur in the future. Such events, however, offer only a very partial perspective on the wider picture in terms of the proportion these acts form of the overall number of homicides which take place, whilst exerting a disproportionate influence on public attitudes and, indeed, the political agenda. Additionally, they deflect attention from the very real risks faced by people experiencing mental illness in terms of suicide and self-harm, the risk of neglect and abuse from others, the experience of stigma and prejudice and the risks that may be associated with using mental health services, including loss of liberty and **iatrogenic** damage from pharmacological and other forms of treatment.

Iatrogenic of illness that is caused by medical treatment intended to relieve symptoms.

It is relevant here to examine briefly some of the evidence regarding the risk to others posed by people with mental illness, much of which has been gathered by the National Confidential Inquiry into Suicide and Homicide by People with Mental Illness, based at the University of Manchester. Figures for the period January 1997 to December 2005 found that of a total of 5,189 homicide offences in England and Wales, only 10 per cent of the perpetrators had had contact with mental health services in the previous twelve months. At a time when the general homicide rate in the population rate has been seen to be increasing, the rate of homicides by mental health patients has been seen to decline from the mid-1970s onwards, with commentators noting that this may be due to improvements in treatment and services, as well as that changes in the categorization and recording of related information may have had some impact (Large et al., 2008). At the same time there is some suggestion of an increase in homicides committed by people with a mental illness who are outside of the mental health services and who have not been patients (National Confidential Inquiry into Suicide and Homicide by People with Mental Illness, 2009a: 36). Research into homicides in four high-income countries (Nielssen et al., 2009) also found that stranger homicide committed by people with psychosis is extremely rare, and even rarer when patients have received treatment with anti-psychotic medication. This study concluded that the low numbers and lack of distinguishing characteristics associated with such events rendered risk assessment of little assistance, although homelessness and the presence of anti-social behaviour were seen to feature in some incidents.

It is also perhaps significant to note that, whilst the numbers of people admitted to hospital has declined over recent years, the proportion of those who are compulsorily detained is increasing. A total of 47,600 detentions were made under the Mental Health Act in 2007–8, of which 28,100 were formal admissions to hospital, with the remaining 19,500 being formally detained after originally being admitted to hospital on a voluntary basis. This represents a slight increase over the previous year and an increase of 2,685 over the 1997–8 total (NHS Information Centre, 2008b). It is inevitable that these figures reflect a situation where concerns regarding the severity of the condition and any associated risk issues will be more likely to figure prominently.

The case of Benjamin Holiday, a 23-year-old man with a diagnosis of paranoid schizophrenia who killed a pregnant woman unknown to him, Tina Stevenson, in the street near her home in 2005, offers an example of a homicide inquiry with associated lessons and recommendations, as well as highlighting the difficulties of reviewing events with hindsight. Holiday pleaded not guilty to murder but guilty to manslaughter on the grounds of diminished responsibility. An external report (Dale et al., 2008) agreed with the main findings of the internal investigation, which were that Holiday's carers were not routinely consulted and that risk assessments were limited and failed to note the patient's full history and the sequence of events leading up to his previous hospital admission before the murder took place, with the added comment that risk assessment documentation was not used to its full potential. Crucially, the report states that 'There was no record that risk issues were routinely discussed at the inpatient multi-disciplinary team meetings and they did not appear to have been fully taken into account' (2008: 5). It was acknowledged that Holiday was difficult to engage and did not fully comply with his medication. Despite concerns regarding substance abuse and possible drug-induced psychosis, this was not comprehensively explored and a carer's assessment had not taken place. The role of the Approved Social Worker (ASW) in not making an application for admission the previous year is specifically mentioned as a missed opportunity, given the previous history of Holiday's improvement when under section. Additionally, his mother was not given information about her rights as the nearest relative. The report concludes that the case of Holiday was one of 'under treatment' and that his care should have been more assertively managed. Holiday is now detained indefinitely at a special hospital.

Despite some clear messages from a report such as this, it is also important to recognize the shortcomings of a review based on hindsight. The Royal College of Psychiatry's Report on risk states that:

> Risk, however, cannot be eliminated. Accurate prediction is never possible for individual patients. While it may be possible to reduce risk in some settings, the risks posed by those with mental disorders are much less susceptible to prediction because of the multiplicity of, and complex interrelation of, factors underlying a person's behaviour.
>
> (2008: 9)

Furthermore, as Stanley and Manthorpe (2001: 78) point out, the reading of risk inquiries, whilst helpful in many respects, also requires caution, as 'Hindsight allows us to weave causal patterns which may not have existed between omissions of care and the act of homicide.' In the example of Holiday, it is possible that, had the ASW decided to apply for compulsory admission the previous year, it might not have been successful in preventing the homicide and might have increased Holiday's disengagement with services. For the ASW concerned, the judgement was also influenced by the complex decision-making required for an application for detention, including the requirement to take the 'least restrictive alternative'.

Reports such as this can also be seen as having the purpose of allaying public anxiety as much as contributing significantly to service improvements. Furthermore, the time delay – in this case, four years between the events that took place and the report of the independent inquiry – means that services will already have undergone considerable change. At the same time, despite the many concerns regarding the way in which inquiries into homicides have been addressed within the media and the wider public and policy arena, it is important not to overlook the key messages and themes which consistently reappear in the wake of such events. These can be summarized as:

- failure to obtain sufficient knowledge about the service user's history and to involve carers;
- poor record-keeping and communication between disciplines;
- lack of interagency collaboration;
- ineffective assessment and management of risk.

Integrating Risk Assessment and Management into Practice

Prevailing approaches to risk assessment and management are frequently experienced by service users as disempowering and stigmatizing, focusing almost exclusively on risk avoidance and in isolation from issues of recovery. However, there are various positive ways in which service users and carers can be involved in addressing risk in a more inclusive and enabling fashion. This can include the use of crisis planning and advance directives, which build on the wishes and experiences of service users and carers in determining how they are to be supported and treated if they become unwell in the future and are not able to make decisions.

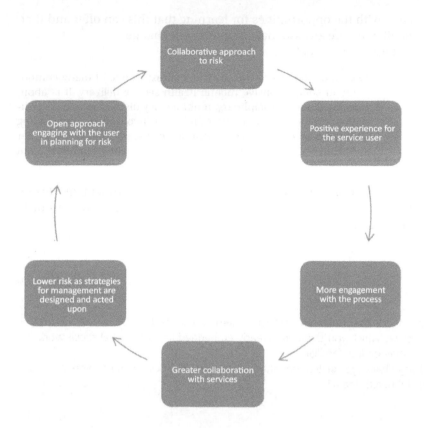

Figure 11.1   Collaborative risk management
Source: Department of Health (2007: 12)

A model of collaborative risk management can be found in *Best Practice in Managing Risk* (Department of Health, 2007: 12), which offers an alternative to a defensive cycle that can develop in working with service users (see Figure 11.1).

Reflection point

Consider issues of risk assessment and management from the perspective of a service user.
   What are the messages that you would want to give a social worker about the things that they could do that would be helpful in building a collaborative and positive approach?

Embedding risk assessment in the process of care planning also offers the opportunity to consider risk from a broader perspective including, for example, the risk of social exclusion or poor housing. The idea of positive risk-taking is also essential in promoting recovery, recognizing that people can make their own choices and decisions. All too often the right to fail is denied to users of mental health services, along with the opportunities for learning that this can offer and that, for all of us, are an essential component of change.

Morgan writes that:

> risk should be placed into its true context as one of many components in comprehensive mental health service delivery. It is about integrated, multi-disciplinary, multi-agency discussion and co-ordination; promoting service user and carer involvement, and valuing colleagues across all sectors. Risk is an integral part of the wider spectrum of good mental health care, and of health promotion ... not separate from it!
>
> (2000: 7)

Guidance from the Department of Health (Department of Health, 2007) summarizes sixteen best practice points, which are set out in Figure 11.2.

Activity

Read through the points for best practice in risk management (Figure 11.2).

Highlight any key issues which you think are already embedded in professional social work practice and any that may be less familiar.

Can you think of any challenges or tensions that might arise for social workers working in a multidisciplinary mental health team?

Social Work and the Role of the Approved Mental Health Professional

Despite the changes introduced by the 2007 Mental Health Act, social workers continue to make a major contribution when it comes to situations of assessment where risk is involved. Those social workers with ASW status at the point of the new act being implemented were effectively transformed into Approved Mental Health Professionals (AMHPs) overnight, and as yet there is no evidence of a large influx of other professionals taking on this work. This may change over time, as one of the barriers to change is not so much the availability of interest from the other eligible professional groups, but a range of organizational and professional issues regarding responsibility for the authorization and funding of training for AMHPs. This currently remains with the local authorities and includes concerns regarding the impact on pay and conditions for the various professional groups involved. It is likely that attempts to reconcile these various interests between local authorities and health trusts may take some time to resolve. For social workers, there is also some anxiety that, despite their experience, other professional groups taking on AMHP responsibilities may be rewarded more favourably.

1. Best practice involves making decisions based on knowledge of the research evidence, knowledge of the individual service user and their social context,knowledge of the service user's own experience, and clinical judgement.

Fundamentals:
2. Positive risk management as part of a carefully constructed plan is a required competence for all mental health practitioners.
3. Risk management should be conducted in a spirit of collaboration and basedon a relationship between the service user and their carers that is as trustingas possible.
4. Risk management must be built on a recognition of the service user'sstrengths and should emphasise recovery.
5. Risk management requires an organisational strategy as well as efforts by the individual practitioner.

Basic ideas in risk management:
6. Risk management involves developing flexible strategies aimed at preventing any negative event from occurring or, if this is not possible, minimising the harm caused.
7. Risk management should take into account that risk can be both general and specific, and that good management can reduce and prevent harm.
8. Knowledge and understanding of mental health legislation is an important component of risk management.
9. The risk management plan should include a summary of all risks identified, formulations of the situations in which identified risks may occur, and actions to be taken by practitioners and the service user in response to crisis.
10. Where suitable tools are available, risk management should be based on assessment using the structured clinical judgement approach.
11. Risk assessment is integral to deciding on the most appropriate level of risk management and the right kind of intervention for a service user.

Working with service users and carers:
12. All staff involved in risk management must be capable of demonstrating sensitivity and competence in relation to diversity in race, faith, age, gender, disability and sexual orientation.
13. Risk management must always be based on awareness of the capacity for the service user's risk level to change over time, and a recognition that each service user requires a consistent and individualised approach.

Individual practice and team working:
14. Risk management plans should be developed by multidisciplinary and multiagency teams operating in an open, democratic and transparent culture that embraces reflective practice.
15. All staff involved in risk management should receive relevant training, which should be updated at least every three years.
16. A risk management plan is only as good as the time and effort put into communicating its findings to others.

Figure 11.2   Best practice points for managing risk
Source: Department of Health (2007: 5–6)

Notwithstanding these issues, early and anecdotal feedback from AMHP training where nurses have been involved indicate that there is a greater level of shared values and perspectives between the different professions than was initially anticipated. As yet there is little evidence for concerns regarding the potential for health practitioners to be less independent or impartial in response to their medical colleagues, in response to traditional professional roles and expectations or as a result of being employed within the same organization. In reality the location of social workers in health settings and community mental health teams can lead to the development of a primary sense of allegiance to the interprofessional team rather than the wider social work community or the local authority, and this in itself has the potential to create different pressures and dynamics regarding their independence. Additionally, in some areas, the creation of Joint Care Trusts has also challenged the traditional health and social care divide.

The continuing role of the local authority as well as the General Social Care Council in the accreditation of training for AMHP responsibilities, however, acts to reinforce the importance of a social work perspective in this area of work. This extends beyond the role of the AMHP in making an application for compulsory admission to hospital and includes being involved in decisions regarding compulsory treatment orders and the preparation of reports for Mental Health Review Tribunals. Experienced mental health professionals, including social workers, are also eligible for new roles such as **Approved Clinician**. The implications of proposals to transfer the professional regulation of social work to a newly configured Health Professions Council remain to be seen (Community Care, 2010).

Approved Clinician position for which registered occupational therapists and social workers, first level mental health and learning disability nurses, chartered psychologists and doctors can now be approved, subject to various training and competence requirements. This role includes powers to detain a patient for up to seventy-two hours and writing reports for patients involved in criminal proceedings or under sentence. They are then eligible to take on the role of Responsible Clinician (see Chapter 4).

Specific Areas of Mental Health Social Work Practice Involving Risk

Responding to issues of suicide, self-harm, neglect and abuse

The importance of considering all aspects of risk within the wider framework of the Care Programme Approach (CPA) has already been discussed earlier in this chapter, recognizing that service users can be victims of neglect, abuse, exploitation and exclusion as well as vulnerable to suicide and self-harm.

Evidence relating to the suicide of people in contact with mental health services showed that 26 per cent of the 50,352 suicides committed between January 1997 and December 2006 involved people who had been in contact with mental health services in the previous twelve months. The majority of these suicides occurred outside of an in-patient setting. As with the general population the rate is seen to be in decline, as were those instances of suicide preceded by non-compliance with treatment or contact with services. The Inquiry Report (National Confidential Inquiry into Suicide and Homicide by People with Mental Illness, 2009a) does, however, draw attention to the 1 per cent of all patient suicides which were committed by people with eating disorders, the majority of whom are women. A number of risk factors have been associated with the risk of suicide (Department of Health, 2007) and are listed in Figure 11.3.

The following activity returns to Sharon, whose time line was introduced in Chapter 10, and offers an opportunity to consider how critical and reflective social work practice may contribute to working with someone at risk of self-harm.

Activity

Revisit Sharon's time line in Chapter 10 and list the various ways in which Sharon may be vulnerable to risk.

Think about how these experiences may limit Sharon in the future and how they could be overcome.

Demographic factors	Male
	Increasing age
	Low socio -economic status
	Unmarried, separated, widowed
	Living alone
	Unemployed
Background history .	Deliberate self -harm (especially with high suicide intent)
	Childhood adversity (e.g. sexual abuse)
	Family history of suicide
	Family history of mental illness
Current 'context'	Suicidal ideation
	Suicide plans
	Availability of means
	Lethality of means
Clinical history	Mental illness diagnosis (e.g. depression, bipolar disorder, schizophrenia)
	Personality disorder diagnosis (e.g. borderline personality disorder)
	Physical illness, especially chronic conditions and/or those associated with pain and functional impairment (e.g. multiple sclerosis, malignancy, pain syndromes)
	Recent contact with psychiatric services
	Recent discharge from psychiatric inpatient facility
Psychological and psychosocial factors	Hopelessness
	Impulsiveness
	Low self -esteem
	Life event
	Relationship instability
	Lack of social support

Figure 11.3 Risk factors associated with suicide
Source: Department of Health (2007)

It is likely that your list will include a number of different issues including the risk of self-harm if Sharon continues to overdose when she is distressed, or even the risk of killing herself in response to her voices. You may also have considered the risks associated with her prescribed medication or of further admissions to hospital, particularly if this were as a result of being 'sectioned' under the Mental Health Act. There are also risks relating to poverty, poor housing and exploitation, as well as others that you may have identified.

People with dangerous and severe personality disorders and mentally disordered offenders: secure and forensic work

Forensic work takes place at the interface between the mental health and criminal justice systems and services, with high levels of mental health difficulties found within the prison population. Figures indicate that 70 per cent of prisoners have two or more mental health problems (Singleton et al., 1998) and that over half of prisoners experience common mental health problems (Sainsbury Centre for Mental Health, 2008). Research by O'Brien et al. (2003) estimated a prevalence rate for neurotic disorders amongst women prisoners of 66 per cent, compared to 16 per cent in the general population, and high levels of self-harm, with 50 per cent of women prisoners having experienced physical or sexual abuse. The plight of women in the criminal justice system is recognized both nationally and internationally as an area of concern (Home Office, 2007; WHO, 2009b).

Levels of mental health problems are also especially high amongst those detained under the Imprisonment for Public Protection provision of the Criminal Justice Act 2003, which enables an indeterminate sentence to be passed on those offenders whose offences do not carry a life sentence but who are seen by the courts as dangerous. Once released such prisoners are on a life licence and subject to recall if the licence terms are breached. The lack of a definite release date and the uncertainty of an indeterminate sentence are themselves stressful and likely to affect mental health, with no guaranteed access to mental health support such as talking therapies (Sainsbury Centre for Mental Health, 2008). The New Horizons policy (Department of Health/HM Government, 2009) draws on the recommendations of the Bradley Review of people with mental health problems or learning disabilities in the criminal justice system (Bradley, 2009), addressing issues at each and every stage of the process from early intervention, arrest and prosecution through court, prison and community sentences to resettlement, stressing the importance of the design and delivery of co-ordinated services involving partnership working between health, criminal justice and social care agencies.

Forensic mental health services provide hospital and community-based care for mentally disordered offenders, that is, those people who have been charged or sentenced through the courts and where prison is not seen to be appropriate to meet their mental health needs or where, as in the majority of cases, people are transferred from prison to forensic services. Forensic services are designated as high, medium or low secure and there are approximately 4,500 secure places in high and medium secure units (Rutherford & Duggan, 2007). The three high secure units for England and Wales are Ashworth, Broadmoor and Rampton NHS Hospitals, with one in Scotland (Carstairs Hospital). Medium secure units are provided by both NHS and independent sector providers. Low secure beds may also be used for voluntary patients and are frequently used to provide a step-down stage for patients from medium secure units prior to discharge.

The majority of patients in these settings are male, and figures from the Count Me In census (Care Quality Commission, 2010) indicate that White British, Indian and Bangladeshi patients were less likely than average to be on medium or high secure wards, whereas Black Caribbean, Black African, mixed White/Black African and White Irish patients were more likely than average to be on these wards.

Although small numbers of convicted people may stay in forensic services for many years, over half stay for under five years and a third leave within two years. One in five remains there for between five and ten years. Discharge from forensic services is frequently back into the community, although other people remain in hospital or return to prison. Reoffending rates are seen to be very low for those discharged from secure units when compared with people released from prison, and figures include a 2 per cent reoffending rate for violent or sexual offences, compared to 27 per cent and 46 per cent reoffending rates for prisoners released from prison back into the community, for violent and sexual offences respectively (Sainsbury Centre for Mental Health, 2007).

Specialist posts in hospital units enable social workers, usually AMHPs, to contribute to the multiprofessional team discussion, which includes risk assessment and management plans. The role also involves liaison with families and arrangements for rehabilitation and discharge into the community or less secure settings. Close collaboration with other professionals and agencies is likely to involve Multi-Agency Public Protection Arrangements (MAPPA) and the consideration of issues of adult and child protection as well as victim liaison services.

Activity

Mervyn is 42 and has spent the past four years in a medium secure unit. He has a diagnosis of anti-social personality disorder accompanied by depression and a history of petty crime. He was made subject to a hospital order (Section 37) following a serious attack on his ex-girlfriend.

The team on the unit are generally positive about the progress that Mervyn has made and believe that his time with them has provided him with a period of stability in his living environment and his relationships with staff. When he was first admitted his behaviour was challenging; he was confrontational with other patients and very demanding of attention from nurses on the ward. This was addressed by the various members of the multiprofessional team working together to ensure a consistent response to Mervyn's demands and behaviour.

Mervyn's father died some years ago but during his time in hospital his mother has been in regular contact. He has had virtually no contact with an older sister who was a close friend of his ex-girlfriend.

Mervyn is now working towards discharge into the community and is eventually hoping to be housed in the area where his mother is still living and where he grew up. In the first instance he is moving to supported accommodation as part of a phased plan for living independently.

List the agencies that might need to be involved in planning for Mervyn's return to the community.

What are some of the issues that might need to be considered in relation to Mervyn's discharge from hospital?

Jerome, the social worker who is co-ordinating the work with Mervyn, is based within the multiprofessional team and has already had some contact with Mervyn on the hospital ward. Jerome is aware that Mervyn's plan to return to his local community raises some very particular challenges that will have to be addressed. Jerome is especially concerned to take an integrated and holistic approach to balancing issues of risk and recovery and is concerned that Mervyn's own needs and wishes are not sidelined as a consequence of people's responses to his diagnosis. Jerome is also anxious to ensure that, as far as possible, services and support can be co-ordinated to provide the stability and continuity that have been found to be helpful for Mervyn.

Jerome's plan of action includes the following areas:

- building a relationship with Mervyn and working to promote his interests and wishes;
- co-ordinating services to support Mervyn in the community;
- working with Mervyn's family;
- addressing issues of risk.

In talking with Mervyn, Jerome attempts to be realistic and honest about the level of concern that he is likely to encounter, whilst maintaining a positive attitude. Together they discuss some of the potential challenges that might arise including how Mervyn might deal with any setbacks. Mervyn's own goals include having his own flat and continuing to develop his IT skills, although he is unsure as to whether or not he could initially cope with employment. There is the chance that Mervyn might also be vulnerable to comments in the street or other forms of abuse and harassment which could jeopardize his progress, especially if his history becomes known within the local community. Jerome is concerned that Mervyn could find himself in a cycle of behaviour that could potentially place him and others at risk and, at the very least, disrupt the co-ordination of support and services.

The list of services and people that Jerome sees as likely to be involved is mapped out in Figure 11.4. Jerome is aware that it will be important that everyone involved is regularly informed and updated about Mervyn's support plan. He sets up an agreement that key people from each agency will communicate with one another and also makes sure that Mervyn is aware of this, to counter the possibility that he will move from one agency to another with conflicting accounts of what is happening.

In terms of risk, the particular concerns relate to Mervyn's developing a relationship with a new partner, where his history indicates that he is more likely to resort to violence if there are difficulties. In line with a collaborative approach to risk management, this is shared with Mervyn and he is involved in considering his responses to various scenarios that could potentially develop. Continuing contact

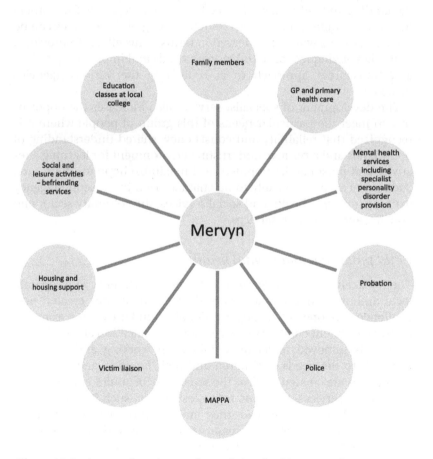

Figure 11.4   A map of services and people involved in Mervyn's support plan

with the psychologist he has been working with for the past eighteen months is seen to be important in identifying issues at an early stage and acting to reduce any possible risks. This is also linked to a relapse prevention plan which is drawn up by Jerome in close collaboration with Mervyn and, with Mervyn's knowledge, is shared with others involved in his care.

In Jerome's experience, there can sometimes be conflicting views regarding confidentiality in situations of this kind. This can also extend to family members as, whilst Mervyn's mother potentially sees herself as a carer, this is not necessarily Mervyn's view and their relationship has not always gone smoothly. Jerome realizes that it will be important to acknowledge the needs of Mervyn's mother as a potential carer, including a carer's assessment, whilst not overstepping the boundaries of confidentiality that Mervyn may wish to maintain. Information regarding Mervyn's conviction will also need to be disclosed to other services involved as well as any potential new partner in the future.

Working with anyone seen to have a personality disorder is often demanding and difficult, not helped by a cycle of rejection from others involved, including services. An understanding of these issues can be seen in Jerome's work with Mervyn in terms of his efforts to provide a non-stigmatizing response to Mervyn's needs and in providing a clear and transparent approach to co-ordinating the various agencies involved.

The development of specialist services also increases the opportunity to meet the particular needs of this group of people where it is recognized that reliability and consistency, shared understanding of boundaries and a positive and trusting environment for learning, creativity and personal development will maximize hope for the future. Such services are also likely to be characterized by close interagency working involving health and social services, the voluntary sector and housing and probation services.

Child protection and mental health

The replacement of generic social services departments with separate local authority children's and adults' departments has created new challenges, as one set of organizational boundaries – for example, between different children's services, such as education and social services – is removed to facilitate joined-up working and a holistic response to the needs of children and their families, and other new boundaries are created, such as the separation of adults' and children's social work services. However, regardless of how such boundaries are constructed and experienced, they are an inevitable part of multi-agency working, and skill is necessary to negotiate and work effectively across these divisions (Roaf, 2002). This is an area of crucial importance in turning our attention to issues of mental health and child protection.

An analysis of serious case reviews in England between 2005 and 2007 (Brandon et al., 2009) examined all the local inquiries into situations where a child died or was seriously injured and where abuse or neglect was known or suspected. Out of a total of 189 reviews of cases, in which two thirds of the children died and one third were left seriously injured, nearly three quarters lived with either past or current experience of domestic violence, parental mental ill health or parental substance misuse, and these three factors were often found to co-exist. Depression in one parent or carer was found to feature in over a quarter of the cases, and over two thirds of the children involved had lived with a parent or carer who had past or present experience of mental illness. The report emphasized that the presence of mental ill health or other factors cannot be seen to predict the chance of a child being harmed or killed. However, in the context of families who are overwhelmed with difficulties, such factors must be considered as increasing the risks to the children involved.

The report refers to situations involving young babies and where a number of agencies were involved. In one example, child care issues were recorded as not relevant by a mental health worker in a case where the lodger, who had been assessed, went on to injure the child fatally (Brandon et al., 2009: 47). It is also worth noting that the inquiry into the death of Baby P., a 17-month-old boy whose mother and her partner were convicted of his murder in 2007, highlighted the involvement of mental health agencies alongside other health and social work organizations and that these were seen to be ineffective in working together on a number of counts (Haringey Local Safeguarding Children Board, 2009). Overall, a number of concerns that are of particular relevance when considering mental health and child protection issues can be identified from this report, and these are summarized in Figure 11.5.

In particular, the first point highlights the delicate balance to be achieved between using a strengths-based approach and managing issues of risk. On the one hand, strengths-based work is generally recognized as being essential for engagement and building collaboration with service users in any area of social work practice, whilst on the other hand, there is a concern that risks to the child or anyone else may not be adequately recognized. In addressing this balance, Brandon et al. call for practitioners to adopt a stance of 'respectful uncertainty' (2009: 114) alongside 'rigorous systematic thinking and analysis' in order for specialist expertise to be pooled to make sense of the complexity of the many factors involved in child protection. Similarly, the National Director for Mental Health in England states in his foreword to the guidance on *Best Practice in Managing Risk* (Department of Health, 2007: 3) that a good therapeutic relationship requires both sympathetic support and an objective assessment of risk. Such a position can also be seen to have wider application in any aspect of risk assessment in relation to mental health.

- A reluctance among many practitioners, including those in mental health services, to make negative professional judgements about a parent, especially where there was some evidence of success in engaging with services on the part of disadvantaged parents, even when the child was the subject of a child protection plan.
- Adult-focused practitioners' failure to recognize the child or children in the family who becomes 'invisible' and whose needs are overlooked. This is also described as 'silo practice' (Brandon et al., 2009: 47), referring to the way in which workers focus on their own particular area of activity and fail to look at the wider issues affecting other family or household members.
- An assumption that someone else is responsible for seeing the child or in contact with the family.
- Poor communication and information sharing between workers and agencies. These practices are seen as detracting from effective risk assessment and management, and are further compromised when individuals and services are under pressure.

Figure 11.5   Concerns regarding child protection and mental health
Source: Brandon et al. (2009)

A literature review on filicide, defined as the killing of a child by a parent, undertaken by the National Confidential Inquiry into Suicide and Homicide by People with Mental Illness (2009b) also draws attention to issues of mental illness in parents. The report states clearly that the majority of parents with a mental health difficulty pose no threat to their children, but explores the range of complex multiple factors which were seen to contribute to situations leading to the death of a child at the hands of a parent. These include those listed in Figure 11.6, but as the report highlights, the incidence of such events is low, risk factors are widespread and risk is difficult to predict and prevent.

A separate report on serious case reviews (Gilbert et al., 2008) found that out of a total of fifty included, fourteen involved a perpetrator with mental health difficulties. The report suggests that long waiting lists for mental health and substance abuse services may have placed strain on the quality of care offered as well as the potential for effective multi-agency working, and recommends a multi-agency approach to providing antenatal and postnatal care for mothers who experience mental health problems from pregnancy onwards. The collaborative involvement of health visitors and other health and social work professionals is encouraged, along with the use of screening tools such as the Edinburgh Postnatal Depression Scale (Cox et al., 1987) and the assessment of suicidal thinking and ideas about harming their child. The potential contribution of support programmes such as the Nurse–Family Partnership to work with first time teenage mothers is also

Parents having children at a young age

Prior contact with social services re child abuse and neglect

Domestic violence

Social disadvantage/financial instability

Single parent and lack of social support

Suicidal ideation – extended to child

Mental illness (depression and psychosis)

Delusions around the child's health and wellbeing

Postpartum disorders

Substance misuse

Figure 11.6   Risk factors for consideration by practitioners working in childcare and mental health services
Source: National Confidential Inquiry into Suicide and Homicide by People with Mental Illness (2009b)

highlighted. There is, however, a risk that interventions such as these are more easily focused on mothers and that attention also needs to be directed towards working with fathers.

The Social Work Contribution to Interprofessional and Multi-Agency Working

A recurring theme throughout this chapter has been the need for joined-up working between practitioners and agencies, and the remainder of the chapter will focus specifically on the challenges and opportunities that are presented to social workers in this area. Reference has already been made in Chapter 3 to the wider policy context within which integrated team working is emphasized as part of the 'modernization' agenda, and this forms the backdrop for the introduction of a number of key issues relating to team working in practice, recognizing that the range of literature and experience in this area is increasing at a rapid rate and that an extensive discussion is beyond the scope of this text.

The language of interprofessional and multi-agency working is itself complex, and a sometimes confusing array of different terms is likely to be encountered both within the literature and in practice. At the heart of interprofessional practice, however, is the idea that working together will promote the most effective outcomes for service users and carers, drawing on a wide range of knowledge and skills, but with a clear sense of common purpose and values. This can also be illustrated by the distinction that has been drawn between a team of experts and an expert team, where there is an emphasis on the individual expertise of each team member in the former as compared to the creation of a shared team culture and purpose associated with the latter (Bleakley et al., 2006).

What promotes effective interprofessional team working?

A number of factors have been identified as helpful in promoting good interprofessional working, including the presence of supportive organizational structures and policies, positive leadership, opportunities for effective communication and team building, and clarity regarding roles and responsibilities (Larkin & Callaghan, 2005; Robinson et al., 2008).

Notwithstanding the wider organizational and structural issues that need to be addressed in order to provide an environment that is conducive to interprofessional working, attention also needs to be paid to the individual, personal qualities and skills of team members, including a positive attitude to joined-up working and a self-reflective approach. There continue to be concerns, however, that different professional roles are not fully understood and valued (Larkin & Callaghan, 2005), potentially leading to ambiguity and confusion and the maintenance of professional tribalism, causing 'silo' practice as referred to in Figure 11.5.

Reflection point

What do you consider to be the skills and knowledge that you have as a social worker that will enable you to make a positive contribution to working with others in an interprofessional mental health team?

How could you help other members of the team to understand the particular contribution of social work?

What could you do to help increase your understanding of the roles and responsibilities of other members of the team?

The term 'communities of practice' has been used by Wenger (1998) to describe the ways in which shared knowledge derived from practice helps to build a sense of community. Such a community requires that people have *mutual engagement* or a sense of belonging; *joint enterprise*, understood as an agreed goal or purpose; and a *shared repertoire* or way of doing things. Associated with this is the notion of a shared language that helps to bridge the gaps that can create obstacles to different professions working together. The concept of bilingualism (Corley & Eades, 2006) may be helpful in negotiating the different values and cultures that may exist in an interprofessional team.

Negotiating the complexities and challenges of working together in teams requires social workers to be both independent and autonomous in their practice, whilst at the same time able to build alliances with others within and outside the team. This is especially important in mental health teams, where social workers may be in a minority compared with other professional colleagues such as nurses and where, in many situations, they may be subject to the requirements of their local authority employer, as well as the Health Trust in which they are based, with resulting differences in pay, conditions and expectations.

Networking and working across agencies

There are more extensive and creative opportunities for joined-up working beyond the setting of the interprofessional team. The emphasis on promoting recovery and social inclusion within the broad policy agenda clearly points to the shared responsibility that exists between government departments, local authorities, the NHS and third sector organizations.

The example of working with Sharon to address risk, explored earlier in this chapter, potentially raises the need to address her housing requirements, leisure activities and physical health care needs. Joining up these systems to produce the most effective package of support for Sharon will require a considered and sensitive approach to ensure that her decisions and preferences remain central to the process.

Working together: what's the point?

In and amongst the many debates regarding working together, it is easy to lose sight of the overall purpose, namely the benefits of effective working for service users and carers. The work of Robinson et al. (2008), although focused primarily on children's services, points to improvements in access to services and a speedier response, better information and communication, increasing involvement and improved outcomes. Hudson (2007: 12) drawing on experience of an integrated adult services team, refers to service users' 'perception of complexity as simplicity' as the best measure of team working.

Within mental health services there have been a number of initiatives to promote Capable Teams in line with the 'New Ways of Working', underpinned by the Ten Essential Shared Capabilities (National Institute for Mental Health in England/Sainsbury Centre for Mental Health Joint Workforce Support Unit, 2004). At the heart of this endeavour is working together with service users and carers to promote recovery.

Concluding Comments

Issues of risk and risk-taking are central to social work and mental health practice, but require critical engagement with the complex issues involved in this uncertain and contested territory. Although this chapter has had to attend to issues of risk with regard to systems of risk assessment and management in order to promote the safety and wellbeing of both service users and others, wider issues of positive risk-taking have also been discussed as a vital ingredient of recovery-focused work.

Onyett writes that 'Without risk there is no change, no development and no learning' (2003: 146). In this sense all aspects of risk need to permeate practice in mental health and must be underpinned by a combination of social work values and attention to principles of social justice and empowerment. Responding to situations of risk and dangerousness, therefore, whilst drawing on appropriate knowledge and skills, requires the continuation of such principles, rather than some kind of special 'magic', and social work practice that works to bring about creative solutions rather than remaining risk-averse.

Working in partnership with service users, carers and other practitioners and agencies within and outside mental health services adds a further layer of complexity to this already multifaceted picture, yet also offers the best opportunities to support service users in working towards their own goals. An approach to practice which is informed by a process of critical reflection will support social workers in making a valuable and effective contribution to the process of interprofessional working and in building and enhancing communication and networks between agencies and systems.

Further Reading

Onyett, S. (2003) *Teamworking in Mental Health*. Basingstoke: Palgrave Macmillan

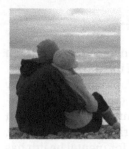

Conclusion

Key points

- The relevance of a mental health perspective in all areas of social work practice
- The value of a social work contribution to mental health, emphasizing a social perspective and issues of social justice
- Building collaborative relationships with service users and carers
- The importance of interprofessional and multi-agency working
- Working with change, contradictions and uncertainty

Introduction

The concluding section of this book will revisit some of the key issues that have been raised in the various chapters. However, in attempting to draw the various strands together, it is important to emphasize that there are not necessarily any clear and unambiguous messages. As in practice, neat and tidy endings are not always possible: instead we are faced with loose ends, unfinished business and a sense of a continuing journey. Despite this, it is still worthwhile to pause and look back, taking the opportunity to reflect on the direction of travel before looking forward to the landscape ahead. This will be addressed by first reviewing the main areas that have been covered in each of the three parts of the book. Second, some of the tensions and contradictions that have been raised will be considered, linked to a discussion regarding the value of a critical and reflective approach to social work practice and mental health and how this may help to sustain the ongoing journey. Finally, some of the potential challenges likely to be encountered in the future will be highlighted.

Looking Back

The four chapters that make up Part 1 of this book have offered a range of perspectives on mental health which together provide an underpinning framework for social work practice. Starting with the voices and experiences of service users and carers emphasized the importance of listening and responding to those whose lives are affected most directly by mental health difficulties, whilst at the same time recognizing that these experiences can, and do, affect many of us personally. Chapter 2 introduced a range of theories, models and concepts that are often encountered when attempting to 'make sense' of mental health issues. The influence of a medical model and the development of psychiatry as well as psychological and sociological perspectives were acknowledged, before considering the significance of current thinking about 'post-psychiatry', a social model of disability, spirituality and recovery. An overview of the policy and legislative context for mental health has been provided within Chapters 3 and 4, locating this within the wider environment of health and social care policy and identifying some of the associated tensions and dynamics.

The two chapters that comprise Part 2 can be seen, in some respects, as representing the heart of the book, in setting out some of the key evidence regarding a social perspective. Chapter 5 addresses issues of inequalities, referring to the social determinants of health and their impact on mental health as they affect both communities and individuals. Particular aspects of diversity, including the mental health of Black and minority ethnic groups and the relevance of gender and sexuality, have been considered in Chapter 6, recognizing the effects of discrimination and oppression on mental wellbeing as well as the ways in which the social construction of mental illness has been instrumental in the labelling of certain groups as deviant or abnormal.

Part 3 of the book has placed practice centre stage, with chapters on working with children and families and with older people, as well as with adults experiencing a range of mental health difficulties. In particular, Chapters 7 and 8 have drawn attention to the need for all social workers to recognize mental health issues as integral to their practice, rather than remaining a discrete area of specialism, underlining the idea that 'mental health is everybody's business'. For convenience, Chapters 9 and 10 have made a somewhat arbitrary distinction between different mental health conditions, including depression and anxiety, personality disorder and psychosis. A clear theme that runs throughout these chapters is the recognition of the significance of life experience, including loss, trauma and abuse, in the development and management of mental health difficulties. Alongside an emphasis on engagement and building relationships, cognitive behavioural therapy and psychosocial interventions have been introduced, as, despite some criticisms, these are likely to be encountered as dominant modes of intervention. Although issues of risk and interprofessional working are addressed at points earlier in the book, these have been brought to the foreground in the final chapter, partly in response to the evidence from various inquiries which have highlighted the need for effective communication and co-ordination between agencies and professionals in managing risk. Maintaining a collaborative approach with service users and carers and working to address positive risk-taking as well as the risks to, rather than from, service users are also important themes.

Tensions and Contradictions

A number of issues will be considered here, beginning with the challenge inherent in this text. This is the challenge of providing a broad introduction to social work and mental health practice that recognizes the multiplicity of views and approaches that are likely to be encountered, whilst at the same time taking a critical stance from a social work perspective. As found by many social workers working in multidisciplinary teams, it can sometimes be hard to see the dividing line between the contribution of social work and that of the other professions involved. Indeed, to some extent, this process is being encouraged with the emphasis on flexible team working and core mental health competences and values, such as those set out in the Ten Essential Shared Capabilities (National Institute for Mental Health in England/Sainsbury Centre for Mental Health Joint Workforce Support Unit, 2004). Whilst in practice the increasing blurring of boundaries may be an essential part of working with other professionals and practitioners, this inevitably raises questions regarding the unique contribution of social work.

This is further complicated by the increasing acceptance of interactional and multifactorial models that recognize the part played by social as well as psychological and biological factors in mental well-being. Superficially it may appear that social work experience and knowledge, embedded within an understanding of the importance of social relationships, the wider environment and the nature of power and inequalities, is now an integral part of the repertoire of all mental health practitioners. One response might be to understand this as a process of colonization, as what was previously considered to be the territory of social work is now claimed by others. An alternative response might be to recognize the dynamic and constantly changing nature of what is seen to be knowledge, created and re-created in the lived experiences of mental health survivors and service users as well as practitioners. As suggested in the Introduction, we need to seek out common ground in order to move theory and practice forward, recognizing that there is no *one* truth.

Related to this are the tensions in the prevailing emphasis on evidence-based practice, raising questions about exactly what counts as evidence and how this is interpreted. All too often, this is exclusively focused on empirical research generated within a positivist and quantitative paradigm, relegating qualitative and constructivist approaches, including service user experiences, to the sidelines. As Frost cautions: 'A dogmatic adherence to evidence-based practice immediately dismantles the possibility of any partnership working with service users' (2002: 50). At the same time, however, there is a need to test out the effectiveness of new and innovative approaches to practice, including both individual and service level interventions.

A further challenge can be found in the broader discussion of the impact of social inequalities and their impact on mental health, considered in the middle part of this book. Despite the increasing attention being paid to such issues and their recognition within the wider debates on public health, there is a continuing lack of congruence between the evidence and the interventions that are offered. The latter frequently remain focused on individual lifestyle choices and notions of personal responsibility, couched in terms of 'co-production' of health, rather than addressing deep-rooted aspects of disadvantage and inequality. Equally there is a need to avoid casting individuals as helpless victims of circumstance, instead identifying the many and varied strategies that are creatively deployed to resist adversity and ensure survival.

Tensions also exist within the current political and organizational environments in which practice takes place, in both statutory and non-statutory settings. The drive to implement managerial practices within a target-setting culture acts to prioritize technical and procedural processes at the expense of professional practices and decision-making. Examples of this may be found in the introduction of call centres as a first point of contact and an understanding of 'care' as a commodity to be packaged and delivered, rather than as a process based on relationship. Working with people who are experiencing mental health difficulties and whose experience of services may not always have been positive requires social workers to have the capacity – and the time – for 'being', not simply 'doing' (Keeping, 2008).

Critical reflection in social work

The various issues highlighted in the previous section point to a complex and uncertain terrain to be navigated with care and consideration. However, whilst managing uncertainty has been viewed as a key feature of professional social work, social work values and a concern for social justice can also be seen to offer a firm foundation for practice, providing an anchor amidst complexity. Critical reflection also provides a means of unpicking or 'deconstructing' practice, opening up new ways of understanding and thinking. This is particularly salient at a time when managerial and organizational imperatives are experienced as a threat to the exercise of professional judgement and decision-making. Bolton writes, with regard to the prevailing culture, that reflective practice is, 'a supported process which allows, encourages even, doubt and uncertainty [and] paradoxically gives [professionals] strength in the face of such attempts to control. In order to retain political and social awareness, professional development work needs to be rooted in the public and the political as well as the private and the personal' (Bolton, 2010: 11).

Throughout the book the importance of building relationships with people experiencing mental health difficulties has been emphasized, regardless of setting. The process of engagement that this requires – being able to respond with empathy and sensitivity – makes demands on the personal as well as the professional resources of the worker. This capacity to manage difficult and complex emotions in its turn requires measured consideration of boundaries and attention to one's own emotional wellbeing. None of this can be managed in isolation, and access to supervision and support is essential. There may be particular issues here for those social workers who are seconded into multiprofessional teams and who may be the sole social worker in their setting. Such situations may offer opportunities to develop shared frameworks within communities of practice (Wenger, 1998), potentially addressing issues of power and inequality, issues that are inextricably tied up with notions of mental health and illness, as explored earlier. Additionally, multiprofessional working may provide a challenging environment within which social workers have to advocate strongly for espousing a social perspective and to challenge injustice.

Looking Forward: The Challenges Ahead

Economic uncertainty and the impact of global and national economic crises provide a challenging environment for developing mental health and social work practice. The drive for 'efficiencies' in the public sector is likely to be accompanied by increasing managerial pressures and a reduction in resources, impacting significantly on social work services. At the same time this environment will impact on the lives of people who are already on the margins, experiencing poverty, inequality and discrimination. As we have seen, this is likely to increase the numbers of those affected by mental health difficulties, with significantly greater and more complex demands being placed on a range of social care and health services. This point was made by Gilbert (2003: 103), who comments that: 'The irony . . . is that social circumstances would seem to make the need for social work even more evident and imperative, and yet social work, at least in its current form and host organization, is often looked at askance.' Reflecting on this point in 2010 would suggest that this imperative is even stronger.

Whilst acknowledging the difficulties that are likely to be encountered, it is also important to consider the strengths and resources that can be drawn on. These can be found within individuals and in groups and teams, and have the potential to increase exponentially when alliances and partnerships are created to offer mutual support in pursuit of common objectives. At the level of practice, this might include building links with service user groups or community organizations to devise creative solutions to problems or to challenge policies or processes that are unjust or discriminatory. Increasing opportunities for the involvement and participation of mental health service users and carers may also create new ways of thinking and responding to health and other inequalities, as well as promoting recovery and social inclusion.

Sharing practice and knowledge across professional and disciplinary boundaries also offers possibilities for innovative practices in responding to complex problems and dilemmas, including questions of risk. This may need to draw on both realist and constructivist ways of thinking about the world, combining, for example, quantitative knowledge about the over-representation of certain groups within mental health statistics with an understanding of the lived experiences of those who are directly involved. It will also be important to respond positively to new opportunities and developments, such as the newly created College of Social Work or the School of Social Care Research, now established within the National Institute for Health Research. Maintaining relationships and communication between social workers engaged in different areas of practice and bridging the gap that often appears between mental health and child care social work, to name just one, is also an essential part of this process.

The creation of new ways of thinking and practice will rely on the necessity of challenging the dichotomous thinking which is often a response to change: it is either rejected or embraced, seen as either negative or positive. Staying hopeful about the future requires us to be able to identify different options and scenarios and choose 'in a planned way between myriad possibilities' (Adams et al., 2009: 7). Despite the complexities and uncertainties that characterize mental health and social work, the principles of social justice and human rights continue to offer a vital 'touchstone' that can inform practice.

References

Acheson, D. (1998) *Independent Inquiry into Inequalities in Health Report*. London: Stationery Office

Ackerman, P. T., Newton, J. E., McPherson, W. B., Jones, J. G. & Dykman, R. A. (1998) Prevalence of post traumatic stress disorder and other psychiatric diagnoses in three groups of abused children (sexual, physical, and both). *Child Abuse and Neglect*, 22(8): 759–74

Adams, R., Dominelli, L. & Payne, M. (2009) *Practising Social Work in a Complex World*. 2nd edn. Basingstoke: Palgrave Macmillan

ADSS (2002) *Deaf Children: Positive Practice Standards in Social Services*. London: ADSS

Allen, R., Gilbert, P. & Onyett, S. (2009) *Leadership for Personalization and Social Inclusion in Mental Health*. London: SCIE

American Psychiatric Association (1994) *Diagnostic and Statistical Manual of Mental Disorders*. 4th edn. Washington, DC: APA

Anthony, W. (1993) Recovery from mental illness: the guiding vision of the mental health service system in the 1990s. *Psychosocial Rehabilitation Journal*, 16(4): 11–23

Antonovsky, A. (1987) *Unraveling the Mystery of Health*. San Francisco: Jossey-Bass

Appignanesi, L. (2008) *Mad, Bad and Sad: A History of Women and the Mind Doctors from 1800 to the Present*. London: Virago

Arnstein, A. (1969) A ladder of citizen participation. *Journal of the American Institute of Planners*, 35(4): 216–24. Reprinted in Gates, R. & Stout, F. (eds) (1996) *The City Reader*. 2nd edn. London: Routledge

Ashworth, A. L. (1975) *Stanley Royd Hospital Wakefield: One Hundred and Fifty Years – A History*. Wakefield: Wakefield District Health Authority

Atkinson, J., Reilly, J., Garner, H. & Patterson, L. (2005) *Review of Literature Relating to Mental Health Legislation*. Edinburgh: Scottish Executive

Audini, B. & Lelliott, P. (2002) Age, gender and ethnicity of those detained under Part II of the Mental Health Act 1983. *British Journal of Psychiatry*, 180: 222–6

Audit Commission (1986) *Making a Reality of Community Care*. London: Stationery Office

Audit Commission (2000) *Forget Me Not: Mental Health Services for Older People*. London: Audit Commission

Bailey, D. (2002) Mental health. In Adams. R., Dominelli, L. & Payne, M. (eds), *Critical Practice in Social Work*. Basingstoke: Palgrave

Baker, P. (1995) *The Voice Inside: A Practical Guide to Coping with Hearing Voices*. Gloucester: Handsell

Balbernie, R. (2001) Circuits and circumstances: the neurobiological consequences of early relationship experiences and how they shape later behaviour. *Journal of Child Psychotherapy*, 27(3): 237–55

Baldwin, N. (2000) *Protecting Children, Promoting Their Rights.* London: Whiting & Birch

Baldwin, N. (2009) Laying the foundations for good health in childhood. In Bywaters, P., McLeod, E. & Napier, L. (eds), *Social Work and Global Inequalities.* Bristol: Policy Press

Baldwin, N. & Walker, L. (2005) Assessment. In Adams, R., Dominelli, L. & Payne, M. (eds), *Social Work Futures.* Basingstoke: Palgrave Macmillan

Barker, I. & Peck, E. (1987) *Power in Strange Places: User Empowerment in Mental Health Services.* London: Good Practices in Mental Health

Barker, I. & Peck, E. (1996) User empowerment: a decade of experience. *Mental Health Review,* 1(4): 5–13

Barker, P. & Buchanan-Barker, P. (eds) (2004) *Spirituality and Mental Health.* London: Whurr

Barnes, J. & Freude-Lagevardi, A. (2003) *From Pregnancy to Early Childhood: Early Interventions to Enhance the Mental Health of Children and Families.* London: Mental Health Foundation. Available at www.mentalhealth.org.uk/publications/?entryid5=42677&p=8, accessed 27 October 2009

Barnes, M. & Bowl, R. (2001) *Taking Over the Asylum.* Basingstoke: Palgrave

Barnett, E. (2000) *Including the Person with Dementia in Designing and Delivering Care: I Need To Be Me.* London: Jessica Kingsley

Barron, J. (2004) *Struggle to Survive: Challenges for Delivering Services on Mental Health, Substance Misuse and Domestic Violence.* Bristol: Women's Aid Federation

Bartholomew, J. B., Morrison, D. & Ciccolo, J. T. (2005) Effects of acute exercise on mood and well-being in patients with major depressive disorder. *Medicine and Science in Sports and Exercise,* 37(12): 2032–3

Bassett, T. & Repper, J. (2005) Travelling hopefully. *Mental Health Today,* November: 16–18

Beck, U. (1992) *Risk Society: Towards a New Modernity.* London: Sage

Bentall, R. (2003) *Madness Explained.* London: Penguin

Beresford, P. (2000) Service users' knowledges and social work theory: conflict or collaboration? *British Journal of Social Work,* 30: 489–503

Beresford, P. (2003) User involvement in research: exploring the challenges. *Nursing Times Research,* 8(1): 36–46

Bhugra, D., Desai, M. & Baldwin, D. (1999) Attempted suicide in West London: rates across ethnic communities. *Psychological Medicine,* 29(5): 1125–30

Bhui, K. & Sachidaran, S. (2003) Should there be separate services for ethnic minority groups? *British Journal of Psychiatry,* 182: 10–12

Bleakley, A., Boyden, J., Hobbs, A., Walsh, L. & Allard, J. (2006) Improving teamwork climate in operating theatres: the shift from multiprofessionalism into interprofessionalism. *Journal of Interprofessional Care,* 20(5): 461–70

Blofeld, J., Sallah, D., Sashidharan, S., Stone, R. & Struthers, J. (2003) *Independent Inquiry into the Death of David Bennett.* Cambridge: Norfolk, Suffolk and Cambridgeshire Strategic Health Authority. Available at http://guardian.co.uk/sys-files/society/documents/2003/02/12/Bennett.pdf, accessed 5 November 2010

Bolton, G. (2010) *Reflective Practice, Writing and Professional Development.* 3rd edn. London: Sage

Boreham, R., Stafford, M. & Taylor, R. (2002) *Health Survey for England 2000: Social Capital and Health.* London: Stationery Office

Bourdieu, P. (1997) The forms of capital. In Halsey, A. H., Lauder, H., Brown, P. & Stuart Wells, S. (eds), *Education, Culture, Economy and Society*. Oxford: Oxford University Press

Bowl, R. (2007) Responding to ethnic diversity: black service users' views of mental health services in the UK. *Diversity in Health and Social Care*, 4: 201–10

Bowlby, J. (1979) *The Making and Breaking of Affectional Bonds*. London: Tavistock

Boxall, K., Dowson, S. & Beresford, P. (2009) Selling individual budgets, choice and control: local and global influences on UK social care policy for people with learning difficulties. *Policy and Politics*, 37(4): 499–516

Brabban, A. & Turkington, D. (2002) The search for meaning: detecting congruence between life events, underlying schema and psychotic symptoms. In Morrison, A. (ed.), *A Casebook of Cognitive Therapy for Psychosis*. London: Psychology Press

Bracken, P. & Thomas, P. (2005) *Postpsychiatry: Mental Health in a Postmodern World*. Oxford: Oxford University Press

Bracken, P., Giller, J. E. & Summerfield, D. (1995) Psychological responses to war and atrocity: the limitations of current concepts. *Social Science and Medicine*, 40(8): 1073–82

Bracken, P., Greenslade, L., Griffin, B. & Smyth, M. (1998) Mental health and ethnicity: an Irish dimension. *British Journal of Psychiatry*, 172: 103–5

Bradford Dementia Group (1997) *Evaluating Dementia Care: The DCM Method*. 7th edn. Bradford: University of Bradford

Bradley, K. (2009) *The Bradley Report: Lord Bradley's Review of People with Mental Health Problems or Learning Disabilities in the Criminal Justice System*. London: Department of Health

Bradshaw, W. (2002) *The Situation and Experiences of Deaf and Hard of Hearing People: Research into Deafness and Employment*. London: RNID

Brandon, D. (2004) Chocolate cakes. In Barker, P. & Buchanan-Barker, P. (eds), *Spirituality and Mental Health*. London: Whurr

Brandon, M., Bailey, S., Belderson, P., Gardner, R., Sidebotham, P., Dodsworth, J., Warren, C. & Black, J. (2009) *Understanding Serious Case Reviews and Their Impact: A Biennial Analysis of Serious Case Reviews 2005–07*. Research Report DCSF-RR129. London: Department for Children, Schools and Families

Bremner, J. & Hillin, A. (1994) *Sexuality, Young People and Care: Creating Positive Contexts for Training, Policy and Development*. London: Russell House

British Heart Foundation (2005) *Depression and Heart Disease: Factfile*. Available at www.bhf.org.uk, accessed 24 February 2010

Brody, E. (1998) *The Search for Mental Health: A History and Memoir of WFMH 1948–1997*. Baltimore: Williams and Wilkins

Brooker, D. (2005) Dementia care mapping (DCM): a review of the research literature. *Gerontologist*, 45(1): 11–18

Brooker, D. (2007) *Person-Centred Dementia Care*. London: Jessica Kingsley

Broverman, I., Broverman, D., Clarakson, F., Rosenkrantz, P. & Vogel, S. (1970) Sex role stereotypes and clinical judgements of mental health. *Journal of Consulting and Clinical Psychology*, 34: 1–7

Brown, G. & Harris, T. (1978) *Social Origins of Depression*. London: Tavistock

Brown, G., Andrews, B., Harris, T., Adler, Z. & Bridge, L. (1986) Social support, self-esteem and depression. *Psychological Medicine*, 16(4): 813–31

Bucknall, O. & Holmes, G. (2001) Relatives and carers. In Newnes, C., Holmes, G. & Dunn, C. (eds), *This is Madness Too*. Ross-on-Wye: PCCS Books

Buckner, L. & Yeandle, S. (2005) *Older Carers in the UK*. Carers UK. Available at www.carersuk.org/Professionals/ResearchLibrary/Profileofcaring/1207234833, accessed 27 August 2010

Bywaters, P., McLeod, E. & Napier, L. (2009) *Social Work and Global Health Inequalities*. Bristol: Policy Press

Callaghan, P. (2004) Exercise: a neglected intervention in mental health care? *Journal of Psychiatric and Mental Health Nursing*, 11: 476–83

Cameron, M., Edmans, T., Greatley, A. & Morris, D. (2003) *Community Renewal and Mental Health*. London: King's Fund

Campbell, P. (1996) The history of the user movement in the United Kingdom. In Heller, T., Reynolds, J., Gomm, R., Muston, R. & Pattison, S. (eds), *Mental Health Matters: A Reader*. Basingstoke: Macmillan

Care Quality Commission (2010) *Count Me In 2009: Results of the 2009 National Census Of Inpatients and Patients on Supervised Community Treatment in Mental Health and Learning Disability Services in England and Wales*. London: Care Quality Commission. Available at www.cqc.org.uk/guidanceforprofessionals/healthcare/allhealthcarestaff/countmeincensus/countmeincensus2009.cfm, accessed 5 November 2010

Carers UK (2007) *Real Change Not Short Change*. Carers UK. Available at www.carersuk.org, accessed 27 August 2010

Care Sector Improvement Partnership/National Institute for Mental Health in England (2007) *Mental Health: New Ways of Working for Everyone*. Progress Report. London: Department of Health

Care Sector Improvement Partnership/Royal College of Psychiatrists/Social Care Institute for Excellence (2007) *A Common Purpose: Recovery in Future Mental Health Services*. London: Social Care Institute for Excellence

Carr, S. (2004) *Has Service User Participation Made a Difference to Social Care Services?* London: SCIE

Carr, S. (2005) 'The sickness label infected everything we said': lesbian and gay perspectives on mental distress. In Tew, J. (ed.), *Social Perspectives in Mental Health*. London: Jessica Kingsley

Carr, S. (2008) *Personalisation: A Rough Guide*. London: SCIE

Cattan, M. (2006) Introduction. In Cattan, M. & Tilford, S. (eds), *Mental Health Promotion: A Lifespan Approach*. Maidenhead: Open University Press/McGraw-Hill

Cattan, M. & Tilford, S. (eds) (2006) *Mental Health Promotion: A Lifespan Approach*. Maidenhead: Open University Press/McGraw-Hill

Chamberlin, J. (1990) The ex-patients' movement: where we've been and where we're going. *Journal of Mind Behaviour*, 11: 323–6

Chan, M. (2008) Return to Alma-Ata. *Lancet*, 372: 865–6

Chesler, P. (1989) *Women and Madness*. Orlando: Harcourt Brace Jovanovich

Children's Workforce Development Council (2009) *Common Assessment Framework for Children and Young People: Practitioners' Guide*. Leeds: CWDC

Cigno, K. (2002) Cognitive-behavioural practice. In Adams, R., Dominelli, L. & Payne, M. (eds), *Social Work: Themes, Issues and Critical Debates*. 2nd edn. Basingstoke: Palgrave

Coid, J., Kirkbride, J., Barker, D., Cowden, F., Stamps, R., Yang, M. & Jones, P. B. (2008) Raised incidence rates of all psychoses among migrant groups. *Archives of General Psychiatry*, 65(11): 1250–8

Coleman, R. (1999) *Recovery: An Alien Concept*. Gloucester: Handsell

Coleman, R. & Smith, M. (1997) *Working with Voices*. Gloucester: Handsell

Commission for Healthcare Audit and Inspection (2005) *Count Me In*. London: Commission for Healthcare Audit and Inspection

Commission on Social Determinants of Health (2008) *Closing the Gap in a Generation: Health Equity through Action on the Social Determinants of Health*. Geneva: WHO

Community Care (2008) Sheffield's Pakistani community helped with mental illness by Enhanced Pathways in Care project. Available at www.communitycare.co.uk/Articles/2008/05/07/108130/Sheffield39s-Pakistani-community-helped-with-mental-illnes-by-Enhanced-Pathways-In-Care.htm, accessed 5 July 2008

Community Care (2010) GSCC to be scrapped. Available at www.communitycare.co.uk/Articles/2010/07/27/114983/GSCC-to-be-scrapped.htm, accessed 27 July 2010

Cooke, A. (2008) Problems associated with the use of the concept 'mental illness'. In Stickley, T. & Bassett, T. (eds), *Learning About Mental Health Practice*. Chichester: John Wiley

Cooklin, A. (2006) Children as carers of parents with mental illness. *Psychiatry*, 5(1): 32–5

Corley, A. & Eades, E. (2006) Sustaining critically reflective practitioners: competing with the dominant discourse. *International Journal of Training and Development*, 10(1): 30–40

Cosis Brown, H. (2008) Social work and sexuality: working with lesbians and gay men – what remains the same and what is different? *Practice*, 20(4): 265–75

Cowden, S. & Singh, G. (2007) The 'user': friend, foe or fetish? A critical exploration of user involvement in health and social care. *Critical Social Policy*, 27(5): 5–23

Cox, J. L., Holden, J. M. & Sagovsky, R. (1987) Edinburgh Postnatal Depression Scale. *British Journal of Psychiatry*, 150: 782–6

Crepaz-Keay, D. (2008) About the National Survivor User Network. *OpenMind*, 149, January/February

Crome, I., & Chambers, P. with Frisher, M., Bloor, R. & Roberts, D. (2009) *The Relationship between Dual Diagnosis: Substance Misuse and Dealing with Mental Health Issues*. Research Briefing. Available at www.scie.org.uk/publications/briefings/files/briefing30.pdf, accessed 5 November 2010

Crossley, N. (2006) *Contesting Psychiatry: Social Movements in Mental Health*. London: Routledge

Dale, C., Rosenberg, M. & Green, P. (2008) *Report of the Independent Investigation into the Care and Treatment of B: SUI Reference 2005/95*. Leeds: Yorkshire and the Humber Strategic Health Authority

Deegan, P. E. (1988) Recovery: the lived experience of rehabilitation. *Psychosocial Rehabilitation Journal*, 11: 11–19

Deegan, G. (2003) Discovering recovery. *Psychiatric Rehabilitation Journal*, 26(4): 368–76

Deegan, P. (1996) Recovery and the conspiracy of hope. Presented at the Sixth Annual Mental Health Services Conference of Australia and New Zealand, Brisbane, September

Department for Children, Schools and Families (2008) *Targeted Mental Health in Schools Project*. Available at http://publications.everychildmatters.gov.uk/default.aspx?PageFunction=productdetails&PageMode=publications&ProductId=DCSF-00784-2008&, accessed 5 November 2009

Department for Constitutional Affairs (2007) *Mental Capacity Act 2005: Code of Practice*. London: Stationery Office

Department for Education and Skills (2004) *Every Child Matters: Change for Children.* London: HMSO

Department of Health (1998) *Modernising Mental Health Services: Safe, Sound and Supportive.* London: Stationery Office

Department of Health (1999a) *Effective Care Co-ordination in Mental Health Services: Modernizing the Care Programme Approach – A Policy Booklet.* London: Department of Health

Department of Health (1999b) *National Service Framework for Mental Health: Modern Standards and Service Models.* London: Stationery Office

Department of Health (1999c) *Patient and Public Involvement in the New NHS.* London: Department of Health

Department of Health (2000) *The NHS Plan: A Plan for Investment, A Plan for Reform.* Cm. 4818–1. London: Stationery Office

Department of Health (2001a) *Making It Happen: A Guide to Delivering Mental Health Promotion.* London: Department of Health

Department of Health (2001b) *National Service Framework for Older People.* London: Department of Health

Department of Health (2001c) *Research Governance Framework for Health and Social Care.* London: Department of Health

Department of Health (2002a) *Mental Health Policy Implementation Guide: Dual Diagnosis Good Practice Guide.* London: Department of Health

Department of Health (2002b) *Women's Mental Health: Into the Mainstream.* London: Department of Health

Department of Health (2002c) *Developing Services for Carers and Families of People with Mental Illness.* London: Department of Health

Department of Health (2004a) *Choosing Health: Making Health Choices Easier.* London: Stationery Office

Department of Health (2004b) *Care Management for Older People with Serious Mental Health Problems.* London: Department of Health

Department of Health (2004c) *The National Service Framework for Children, Young People and Maternity Services.* London: Stationery Office.

Department of Health (2005) *POPP Project Profiles.* Available at www.dh.gov.uk/prod_consum_dh/groups/dh_digitalassets/@dh/@en/documents/digitalasset/dh_4122623.pdf, accessed 11 November 2009

Department of Health (2006) *Our Health, Our Care, Our Say.* London: Department of Health

Department of Health (2007) *Best Practice in Managing Risk: Principles and Evidence for Best Practice in the Assessment and Management of Risk to Self and others in Mental Health Services.* London: Department of Health

Department of Health (2008a) *Code of Practice: Mental Health Act 1983.* London: Stationery Office

Department of Health (2008b) *Refocusing the Care Programme Approach: Policy and Positive Practice Guidance.* London: Department of Health

Department of Health (2009a) *Local Routes: Guidance for Developing Alcohol Treatment Pathways.* London: Department of Health

Department of Health (2009b) *Report of the Standing Committee on Carers, 2007 to 2009.* London: Department of Health

Department of Health/Department for Education and Skills (2006) *Promoting the Mental Health and Psychological Well-Being of Children and Young People: Report on the Implementation of Standard 9 of the NSF for Children, Young People and Maternity Services.* London: Department of Health

Department of Health/HM Government (2009) *New Horizons: A Shared Vision for Mental Health*. London: Department of Health

Department of Health, Social Services and Public Safety (2003) *Promoting Mental Health: Strategy and Action Plan, 2003–8*. Belfast: Department of Health, Social Services and Public Safety

Dixon, L. & Lehman, A. (1995) Family interventions for schizophrenia. *Schizophrenia Bulletin*, 21: 631–43

Doel, M., Carrol, C., Chambers, E., Cooke, J., Hollows, A., Laurie, L., Maskrey, L. & Nancarrow, S. (2007) *Participation: Finding Out What Difference It Makes*. Stakeholder Participation Guide 20. London: SCIE

Dominelli, L. (2007) Human rights in social work practice: an invisible part of the social work curriculum. In Reichert, E. (ed.), *Challenges in Human Rights: A Social Work Perspective*. New York: Columbia University Press

Dooley, D., Prause, J. & Ham-Rowbottom, K. A. (2000) Underemployment and depression: longitudinal relationships. *Journal of Health and Social Behaviour*, 41: 421–36

Double, D. (2002) Redressing the biochemical imbalance. Available at http://www.critpsynet.freeuk.com/doublesep.htmwww.critpsynet.freeuk.com/doublesep.htm, 5 November 2010

Duggan, M. with Cooper, A. & Foster, J. (2002) *Modernising the Social Model in Mental Health: A Discussion Paper*. TOPPS England for SPN. Available at www.spn.org.uk, accessed 5 November 2010

Equalities Review (2006) *The Equalities Review: Interim Report for Consultation*. London: Equalities Review

European Network of (ex-) Users and Survivors of Psychiatry (2009) Aims and objectives. Available at www.enusp.org, accessed 19 November 2009

Falloon, I. R. H. & Graham-Hole, V. (1994) *Comprehensive Management of Mental Disorders*. Buckingham: Buckingham Mental Health Service

Fawcett, B. & Karban, K. (2005) *Contemporary Mental Health: Theory, Policy and Practice*. Abingdon: Routledge

Featherstone, B., Rivett, M. & Scourfield, J. (2007) *Working with Men in Health and Social Care*. London: Sage

Fennell, P. (1996) *Treatment Without Consent: Law, Psychiatry and the Treatment of Mentally Disordered People since 1845*. London: Routledge

Ferguson, I. (2007) Increasing user choice or privatizing risk? The antinomies of personalization. *British Journal of Social Work*, 37(3): 387–403

Fernando, S. (2002) *Mental Health, Race and Culture*. 2nd edn. Basingstoke: Palgrave Macmillan

Finkelstein, V. (1980) *Attitudes and Disabled People*. New York: Work Rehabilitation Fund

Fish, J. (2006) *Heterosexism in Health and Social Care*. Basingstoke: Palgrave Macmillan

Fook, J. (2002) *Social Work: Critical Theory and Practice*. London: Sage

Foresight Mental Capacity and Wellbeing Project (2008) *Final Report: Executive Summary*. London: Government Office for Science

Foster, J. L. H. (2007) *Journeys through Mental Illness: Clients' Experiences and Understandings of Mental Distress*. Basingstoke: Palgrave Macmillan

Foucault, M. (1965) *Madness and Civilisation*. New York: Random House

Foucault, M. (1981) *The History of Sexuality. Vol.1*. Harmondsworth: Penguin

Frame, J. (2000) *Faces in the Water*. London: Women's Press

Friedl, L. (2009) *Mental Health, Resilience and Inequalities*. Copenhagen: WHO

Frost, N. (2002) Evaluating practice. In Adams, A., Dominelli, L. & Payne, M. (eds), *Critical Practice in Social Work*. Basingstoke: Palgrave

Fryer, D. (1995) Labour market disadvantage, deprivation and mental health. *Psychologist*, 8(6): 265–72

Furedi, F. (1997) *Culture of Fear: Risk-Taking and the Morality of Low Expectations*. London: Cassell

Gamble, C. & Brennan, G. (2000) *Working with Serious Mental Illness*. London: Bailliere Tindall

Giddens, A. (1991) *Modernity and Self Identity*. Cambridge: Polity

Giddens, A. (1998) *The Third Way*. Cambridge: Polity

Gilbert, C., Walker, A., Snell, R. et al. (2008) *Safeguarding Children: The Third Joint Chief Inspectors' Report on Arrangements to Safeguard Children*. Ofsted: London

Gilbert, P. (2003) *The Value of Everything: Social Work and its Importance in the Field of Mental Health*. Lyme Regis: Russell House

Gilman, C. Perkins (2009) *The Yellow Wall-Paper, Herland and Selected Writings*. London: Penguin

Glaser, D. (2001) Child abuse and neglect and the brain: a review. *Journal of Child Psychology and Psychiatry*, 41(1): 97–116

Goffman, E. (1961) *Asylums*. Harmondsworth: Penguin

Goldberg, D. & Goodyer, I. (2005) *The Origins and Course of Common Mental Disorders*. Hove: Routledge

Goldberg, D. & Huxley, P. (1992) *Common Mental Disorders: A Bio-Social Model*. London: Routledge

Goodwin, G. M. (2009) *Evidence-Based Guidelines for Treating Bi-Polar Disorder: Revised Second Edition – Recommendations from the British Association for Psychopharmacology*. Available at www.bap.org.uk/pdfs/Bipolar_guidelines.pdf, accessed 30 August 2010

Graham, H. & Power, C. (2004) *Childhood Disadvantage and Adult Health: A Life Course Framework*. London, Health Development Agency

Grant, A., Townend, M., Mulhern R. & Short, N. (2010) *Cognitive Behavioural Therapy in Mental Health Care*. 2nd edn. London: Sage

Green, H., McGinnity, A., Meltzer, H., Ford, T. & Goodman. R. (2005) *Mental Health of Children and Young People in Great Britain, 2004: A Survey by the Office for National Statistics*. Hampshire: Palgrave-Macmillan

Greenberger, D. & Padesky, C. A. (1995) *Mind Over Mood: Change How You Feel By Changing the Way You Think*. New York: Guilford Press

Griffiths, R. (1988) *Community Care: Agenda for Action*. London: Stationery Office

Guardian (2008) Health inequality getting worse, Alan Johnson admits. 9 June

Guardian (2010) Intervening behind closed doors. 31 March

Hannigan, B. (1999) Mental health care in the community: an analysis of contemporary public attitudes towards, and public representations of, mental illness. *Journal of Mental Health*, 8(5): 431–40

Haringey Local Safeguarding Children Board (2009) *Serious Case Review: Baby Peter*. London: Department for Education

Harper, J. (1993) Reaching out: running a staff care service in the aftermath of disaster. In Newburn, T. (ed.), *Working with Disaster: Social Welfare Interventions during and after Tragedy*. Harlow: Longman

Harris, N., Williams, S. & Bradshaw, T. (eds) (2002) *Psychosocial Interventions for People with Schizophrenia*. Basingstoke: Palgrave Macmillan

Harrison, G. & Melville, R. (2010) *Rethinking Social Work in a Global World*. Basingstoke: Palgrave Macmillan

Hawton, K., Rodham, K. Evans, E. et al. (2002) Deliberate self-harm in adolescents: self report survey in schools in England. *British Medical Journal*, 325: 1207–11

Healthcare Commission (2008) *Fifth Annual Survey of Community Mental Health Service Users*. London: Healthcare Commission

Healthcare Commission (2009) *Equality in Later Life: Older People's Mental Health Services – A National Study*. London: Healthcare Commission

Health Education Authority (1997) *Mental Health Promotion: A Quality Framework*. London: HEA

Healthtalkonline (n.d.) Depression. Available at www.healthtalkonline.org/mental_health/depression/Topic/1488, accessed 24 February 2010

Health, Work and Well-Being Programme (2009) *Working our Way to Better Mental Health: A Framework for Action*. Cm. 7756. London: Stationery Office

Herman, J. L. (1992) *Trauma and Recovery*. London: Pandora

Hicks, S. (2009) Sexuality: social work theories and practice. In Adams, R., Dominelli, L. & Payne, M. (eds), *Practising Social Work in a Complex World*. 2nd edn. Basingstoke: Palgrave Macmillan

HM Government (2008) *Carers at the Heart of 21st Century Families and Communities: A Caring System on Your Side, a Life of Your Own*. London: Department of Health

HM Government (2009) *Work, Recovery and Inclusion: Employment Support for People in Contact with Secondary Mental Health Services*. London: National Mental Health Development Unit

Hobson, S. (1998) The ethics of compulsory removal under Section 47 of the 1948 National Assistance Act. *Journal of Medical Ethics*, 24: 38–43

Hoggett, P. (1997) *Contested Communities: Experiences, Struggles, Policies*. Bristol: Policy Press

Holley, T. (2008) A service user's story: the narrative edge – an account of my own illness and the resulting implications for research and training in health and social work and beyond. In *The Narrative Practitioner: Conference Proceedings*. Wrexham: Glyndwr University

Home Office (2007) *The Corston Report: A Review of Women with Particular Vulnerabilities in the Criminal Justice System*. Available at http://webarchive.nationalarchives.gov.uk/+/http://www.homeoffice.gov.uk/documents/corston-report, accessed 5 November 2010

Hothersall, S., Maas-Lowit, M. & Golightly, M. (2008) *Social Work and Mental Health in Scotland*. Exeter: Learning Matters

Howe, D. (2002) Psychosocial work. In Adams, R., Dominelli, L. & Payne, M. (eds), *Social Work: Themes, Issues and Critical Debates*. 2nd edn. Basingstoke: Palgrave

Hudson, B. (2007) Pessimism and optimism in inter-professional working: the Sedgefield Integrated Team. *Journal of Interprofessional Care*, 21(1): 3–15

Hugman, R. (1998) Service users as consumer. In Hugman, R., *Social Welfare and Social Value: The Role of Caring Professions*. London: Macmillan

Humphreys, C. & Thiara, R. (2003) Mental health and domestic violence: 'I call it symptoms of abuse'. *British Journal of Social Work*, 33: 209–26

Hunt, R. & Dick, S. (2008) *Serves You Right: Lesbian and Gay People's Expectations of Discrimination*. London: Stonewall

Independent (2009) Depression costs economy £8.6billion a year. Available at www.independent.co.uk/life-style/health-and-families/health-news/depression-costs-economy-16386bn-a-year-170618.html, accessed 15 February 2010

Ingleby, D. (1985) Professionals as socialisers: the 'psy complex'. In Scully, A. & Spitzer, S. (eds), *Research in Law, Deviance and Social Control, 7*. New York: Jai Press

Inter-Agency Standing Committee, Reference Group on Mental Health and Psychosocial Support (2010) *Guidance Note for Mental Health and Psychosocial Support Haiti Earthquake Emergency Response: January 2010.* Available at www.who.int/mental_health/emergencies/guidance_note_mhpss_haiti.pdf, accessed 19 February 2010

International Association of Schools of Social Work/International Federation of Social Workers (2001) Definition of social work. Available at www.iassw-aiets.org/index.php?option=com_content&task=blogcategory&id=26&Itemid=51, accessed 24 November 2010

International Federation of Social Workers (2008) *IFSW Policy Statement on Health.* Available at http:///www.ifsw.org/p38000081.html, accessed 5 November 2010

Itzen, C. (2006) *Tackling the Health and Mental Health Effects of Domestic and Sexual Violence and Abuse.* London: Department of Health

Johnstone, L. (2000) *Users and Abusers of Psychiatry.* 2nd edn. London: Routledge

Johnstone, L. (2008) Psychiatric diagnosis. In Tummey, R. & Turner, T. (eds), *Critical Issues in Mental Health.* Basingstoke: Palgrave Macmillan

Jones, R. (ed.) (2008) *Mental Health Act Manual.* 11th edn. London: Sweet and Maxwell

Joseph, J. (2004) Schizophrenia and heredity: why the emperor has no genes. In Read, J., Mosher, L. & Bentall, R. (eds), *Models of Madness: Psychological, Social and Biological Approaches to Schizophrenia.* Hove: Bruner Routledge

Kavanagh, D. J. (1992) Recent developments in expressed emotion and schizophrenia. *British Journal of Psychiatry*, 60: 601–20

Kay, H. (1999) *Bright Futures: Promoting Children and Young People's Mental Health.* London: Mental Health Foundation

Kaysen, S. (1995) *Girl, Interrupted.* London: Virago

Keeping, C. (2008) Emotional engagement in social work: best practice and relationships in mental health work. In Jones, K., Cooper, B. & Ferguson, H. (eds), *Best Practice in Social Work: Critical Perspectives.* Basingstoke: Palgrave Macmillan

Kemshall, H. (2002) *Risk, Social Policy and Welfare.* Buckingham: McGraw-Hill/Open University Press

King, M. & Bartlett, A. (1999) British psychiatry and homosexuality. *British Journal of Psychiatry*, 175: 106–13

King, M., Dewey, S. & Fulford, B. (n.d.) More information on Values-Based Practice and the new Mental Health Act. http://old.nimhe.csip.org.uk/~amendmentworkstreams/the-mental-health-act-amending-workstreams/training/onlines-based-practice.htm

King, M. & McKeown, E. (2003) *Mental Health and Social Wellbeing of Gay Men, Lesbians and Bisexuals in England and Wales.* London: UCL/MIND

King, M., Semlyen, J., See Tai, S., Killaspy, H., Osborn, D., Popelyuk, D. & Nazareth, I. (2007) *Mental Disorders, Suicide and Deliberate Self Harm in Lesbian, Gay and Bisexual People.* Leeds: National Institute for Mental Health in England/Care Services Improvement Partnership

Kitson, N. & Thacker, A. (2000) Adult psychiatry. In Hindley, P. & Kitson, N., *Mental Health and Deafness.* London: Whurr

Kitwood, T. (1997) *Dementia Reconsidered.* Buckingham: Open University Press

Knapp, M. & Scott, S. (1998) The impact of psychotherapy on the lifetime cost of childhood conduct disorder. Unpublished report for the Mental Health Foundation

Kraepelin, E. (1913) Dementia praecox. In Kraepelin, E., *Psychiatrie.* 8th edn. Leipzig: Barth. Trans. in part by Barclay, R. M. (1971) *Dementia Praecox and Paraphrenia.* Huntington, NY: Krieger

Kram, M. & Loeb, M. (2007) Mental health in Deaf adults: symptoms of anxiety and depression among hearing and Deaf individuals. *Journal of Deaf Studies and Deaf Education*, 12(1): 1–7

Laing, R. (1965) *The Divided Self*. Harmondsworth: Penguin

Lancashire, S. (1998) KGV(M) Symptom Scale. Unpublished scale. Institute of Psychiatry

Lancet Global Mental Health Group (2007) Scale up services for mental disorders: a call for action. *Lancet*, 370: 1241–52

Large, M., Smith, G., Swinson, N., Shaw, J. & Nielssen, O. (2008) Homicide due to mental disorder in England and Wales over 50 years. *British Journal of Psychiatry*, 193: 130–3

Larkin, C, & Callaghan, P. (2005) Professionals' perceptions of interprofessional working in community mental health teams. Journal of Interprofessional Care 19(4): 338–46

Leader, D. (2008) A quick fix for the soul. *Guardian*, 9 September

Lee, D. & Newby, H. (1983) *The Problem of Sociology*. London: Unwin Hyman

Leff, J. & Vaughan, C. (1981) The role of maintenance therapy and relatives' expressed emotion in relapse in schizophrenia: a two year follow-up. *British Journal of Psychiatry*, 139: 102–4

Lester, H. & Glasby, J. (2006) *Mental Health Policy and Practice*. Basingstoke: Palgrave Macmillan

Levinson, M. (2010) Working with diversity. In Grant, A., Townend, M., Mulhern, R. & Short, N. (2010) *Cognitive Behavioural Therapy in Mental Health Care*. 2nd edn. London: Sage

Lewis, G. & Sloggett, A. (1998) Suicide, deprivation and unemployment. *British Medical Journal*, 7168: 1283–7

Lhussier, M. & Carr, S. M. (2008) Health-related lifestyle advice: critical insights. *Critical Public Health*, 18(3): 299–309

Livingston, G. & Cooper, C. (2004) User and carer involvement in mental health training. *Advances in Psychiatric Treatment*, 10: 85–92

Llewellyn, A., Agu, L. & Mercer, D. (2008) *Sociology for Social Workers*. Cambridge: Polity

Ludermir, A. & Lewis, G. (2003) Informal work and common mental disorders. *Social Psychiatry and Psychiatric Epidemiology*, 39(5): 337–49

MacDonald, G. & O'Hara, K. (1998) *Ten Elements of Mental Health: Its Promotion and Demotion – Implications for Practice*. London: Society of Health Education and Promotion Specialists

McCrone, P., Dhanasiri, S., Patel, A., Knapp, M. & Lawton-Smith, S. (2008) *Paying the Price: The Cost of Mental Health Care in England to 2026*. London: King's Fund

McDaid, S. (2009) An equality of conditions framework for user involvement in mental health policy and planning: evidence from participatory action research. *Disability and Society*, 24(4): 461–74

McFarlane, L. (1998) *Diagnosis: Homophobic*. London: Project for Advice Counselling and Education

McKeith, I. & Fairburn, A. (2001) Biomedical and clinical perspectives. In Cantley, C. (ed.), *A Handbook of Dementia Care*. Buckingham: Open University Press

McKenzie, K. & Harpham, K. (2006) *Social Capital and Mental Health*. London: Jessica Kingsley

McKenzie, K., Whitley, R. & Weich, S. (2002) Social capital and mental illness. *British Journal of Psychiatry*, 181: 280–3

McLaren, S., Jude, B. & McLachlan, A. (2008) Sense of belonging to the general and gay communities as predictors of depression among Australian gay men. *International Journal of Men's Health*, 7(1): 90–9

McManus, S., Meltzer, H., Brugha, T., Bebbington, P. & Jenkins, R. (eds) (2009) *Adult Psychiatric Morbidity in England, 2007*. Leeds: NHS Information Centre. Available at www.ic.nhs.uk/pubs, 27 February 2009

Mackereth, C. & Appleton, J. (2008) Social networks and health inequalities: evidence for working with disadvantaged groups. *Community Practitioner*, 81(8): 23–6

Marmot, M. (2010) *Fair Society, Healthy Lives: The Marmot Review – Strategic Review of Health Inequalities in England, post2010*. Available at www.marmotreview.org, accessed 5 November 2010

Martin, G., Bergen, H. A., Richardson, A. S., Roeger, L. & Allison, S. (2004) Sexual abuse and suicidality: gender differences in a large community sample of adolescents. *Child Abuse and Neglect*, 28(5): 491–503

Means, R. & Smith, R. (1994) *Community Care, Policy and Practice*. Basingstoke: Macmillan

Meltzer, H., & Gatward, R. with Goodman, R. & Ford, T. (2000) *The Mental Health of Children and Adolescents in Great Britain*. London Office for National Statistics/Stationery Office

Meltzer, H., Lader, D., Corbin, T. et al. (2002) *Non-Fatal Suicidal Behaviour Among Adults aged 16–74 in Great Britain*. London: Stationery Office

Mental Health Act Commission (2009) *Coercion and Consent: Monitoring the Mental Health Act 2007–2009*. The Mental Health Act Commission Thirteenth Biennial Report. London: Stationery Office

Mental Health Foundation (2009) *All Things Being Equal: Age Equality in Mental Health Care for Older People in England*. London: Mental Health Foundation

Meyer, I., Dietrich, J. & Schwartz, S. (2008) Lifetime prevalence of mental disorders and suicide attempts in diverse lesbian, gay and bisexual populations. *American Journal of Public Health*, 98(6): 1004–6

Mind (2008) Employers must work on mental health. Available at www.mind.org.uk/news/252_employers_must_work_on_mental_health, accessed 14 April 2010

Mind (2009) *Personalisation in Mental Health: Breaking Down the Barriers – A Guide for Care Coordinators*. London: Mind

Minshull, P. (n.d.) *Age Equality: What Does It Mean For Older People's Mental Health Services?* Guidance Note: Everybody's Business. Integrated Mental Health Services For Older Adults: A Service Development Guide. National Older People's Mental Health Programme/Care Sector Improvement Partnership. Available at http://its-services.org.uk/silo/files/age-equality-guidance-note-pdf.pdf, accessed 31 July 2010

Miranda, J. J. & Patel, V. (2005) Achieving the Millennium Development Goals: does mental health play a role? *PLoS Medicine*, 2(10): e291

Morgan, S. (2000) *Clinical Risk Management: A Clinical Tool and Practitioner Manual*. London: Sainsbury Centre for Mental Health

Morris, N. (2003) Health, well-being and open space: literature review. Available at www.openspace.eca.ac.uk/pdf/HealthWellbeing.pdf, accessed 13 February 2009

Mueser, K. T., Goodman, L. B., Trumbetta, S. L., Rosenberg, S. D., Osher, C., Vidaver, R., Auciello, P. & Foy, D. W. (1998) Trauma and post-traumatic stress disorder in severe mental illness. *Journal of Consulting and Clinical Psychology*, 66(3): 493–9

Mullen, R., Gibbs, A. & Dawson, J. (2006) Family perspective on community treatment orders: a New Zealand study. *International Journal of Social Psychiatry*, 52(5): 469–78

National Confidential Inquiry into Suicide and Homicide by People with Mental Illness (2009a) *Annual Report: England and Wales, July 2009*. University of

Manchester. Available at www.medicine.manchester.ac.uk/psychiatry/research/suicide/prevention/nci, 5 November 2010

National Confidential Inquiry into Suicide and Homicide by People with Mental Illness (2009b) *Filicide: A Literature Review*. University of Manchester. Available at http://medicine.manchester.ac.uk/psychiatry/research/suicide/prevention/nci, 5 November 2010

National Institute for Health and Clinical Excellence (2004) *Self-Harm: The Short Term Physical and Psychological Management and Secondary Prevention of Self-Harm in Primary and Secondary Care*. National Clinical Practice Guideline Number 16. London: British Psychological Society/Royal College of Psychiatrists

National Institute for Health and Clinical Excellence (2005) *Post-Traumatic Stress Disorder (PTSD): Quick Reference Guide*. London: NICE. Available at http://nice.org.uk/nicemedia/pdf/CGO26quickrefguide.pdf, accessed 19 February 2010

National Institute for Health and Clinical Excellence (2006) *Bipolar Disorder: Quick Reference Guide*. London: NICE. Available at http://guidance.nice.org.uk/CG38/QuickRefGuide/pdf/English, accessed 30 August 2010

National Institute for Health and Clinical Excellence (2009a) *Borderline Personality Disorder: NICE Guidelines on Treatment and Management*. London: British Psychological Society and the Royal College of Psychiatrists

National Institute for Health and Clinical Excellence (2009b) *Depression: Treatment and Management of Depression in Adults Including Adults with a Chronic Physical Health Problem – Quick Reference Guide*. London: NICE. Available at www.nice.org.uk/CG91, accessed 6 August 2010

National Institute for Health and Clinical Excellence (2009c) *Schizophrenia: Quick Reference Guide*. London: NHS. Available at www.nice.org.uk, accessed 7 January 2010

National Institute for Health and Clinical Excellence (2010) *Antisocial Personality Disorder: NICE Guidelines On Treatment, Management and Prevention*. London: British Psychological Society and the Royal College of Psychiatrists

National Institute for Health and Clinical Excellence/Social Care Institute for Excellence (2006) *Dementia: Supporting People with Dementia and Their Carers in Health and Social Care*. London: NICE

National Institute for Mental Health in England (2003) *Inside Outside: Improving Mental Health Services for Black and Minority Ethnic Communities in England*. Leeds: Department of Health

National Institute for Mental Health in England (2005a) *Guiding Statement on Recovery*. Leeds: Department of Health

National Institute for Mental Health in England (2005b) *Mental Health and Deafness: Towards Equity and Access*. Leeds: Department of Health

National Institute for Mental Health in England/Sainsbury Centre for Mental Health Joint Workforce Support Unit (2004) *The Ten Essential Shared Capabilities: A Framework for the Whole of the Mental Health Workforce*. London: NIMHE

National Mental Health Development Unit (n.d.) Stockton Dementia Café. Available at www.nmhdu.org.uk/our-work/mhep/later-life/communities-of-interest/stockton-dementia-cafe, accessed 27 August 2010

National Mental Health Development Unit (2009) *National Suicide Prevention Strategy for England: Annual Report on Progress 2008*. Leeds: NMHDU

National Personality Disorder Programme (n.d.) *Ten Things to Know about PD (Personality Disorder)*. Available at www.personalitydisorder.org.uk/what/definitions/index.php, accessed 8 January 2010

National Spirituality and Mental Health Forum (n.d.) Spirituality and mental health. Available at www.spirituality4rum.org, accessed 15 November 2010

NHS Information Centre (2008a) *Mental Health Bulletin.* Available at www.ic.nhs. uk/webfiles/publications/mental%20health/NHS%20specialist%20mental%20 health%20services/MHMDSexperimental200307/Mental%20Health%20 Bulletin.%20Report.pdf, accessed 5 November 2010

NHS Information Centre (2008b) *In-Patients Formally Detained in Hospital under the1983 Mental Health Act and Other Legislation, England 1997–98 to 2007–08.* Available at http://www.ic.nhs.uk/webfiles/publications/mentalhealthkp90/ Inpatients%20formally%20detained%20in%20hospitals%20under%20the%20 Mental%20Health%20Act%201983%20and%20other%20legislation% 20NHS%20trusts%20and%20independent%20hospitals%2020072008%20 bulletin.pdf, 5 November 2010

NHS Information Centre (2010) *Survey of Carers in Households 2009–10 in England: Provisional Results.* Available at www.ic.nhs.uk/webfiles/publications/Social%20 Care/carersurvey0910/Survey_of_Carers_in_Households_2009_10_England_ Provisional_Results_post_publication.pdf, accessed 27 August 2010

Nielssen, O., Bourget, D., Laajasasulo, T., Liem, M., Labelle, A., Hakkane-Nyholm, H., Koenraadt, F. & Large, M. (2009) Homicide of strangers by people with a psychotic illness. *Schizophrenia Bulletin.* Available at http://schizophreniabulletin. oxfordjournals.org/content/early/2009/10/12/schbul.sbp112.full.pdf+html, accessed 5 November 2010

Northern Ireland Executive (2010) McGimpsey launches EQIA for new Mental Capacity Bill and proposals following McDermott case. Press release, 30 July. Available at www.northernireland.gov.uk/news-dhssps-30072010-mcgimpsey-launches-eqia, accessed 23 August 2010

O'Brien, M., Mortimer, L., Singleton, N. & Meltzer, H. (2003) Psychiatric morbidity among women prisoners in England and Wales. *International Review of Psychiatry,* 15(1): 153–7

Office for National Statistics (2003) *The Mental Health of Young People Looked After by Local Authorities in England.* London: Stationery Office

Office for National Statistics (2010) *Statistical Bulletin: Suicide Rates in the United Kingdom, 1991–2008.* Available at www.statistics.gov.uk, accessed 16 April 2010

Office of the Public Guardian (2009). *Making Decisions: A Guide for People who Work in Health and Social Care.* 4th edn. http://www.publicguardian.gov.uk/docs/opg-603–0409.pdf, accessed 16 November 2010

O'Hagan, M. (1999) Realising recovery: six challenges to the mental health sector. Keynote address to Realising Recovery Conference. Mental Health Commission, November

Onyett, S. (2003) *Teamworking in Mental Health.* Basingstoke: Palgrave Macmillan

O'Sullivan, T. (2009) Managing risk and decision-making. In Adams, R., Dominelli, L. & Payne, M. (eds), *Practising Social Work in a Complex World.* Basingstoke: Palgrave Macmillan

Palmer, R., Chaloner, D. & Oppenheimer, R. (1992) Childhood sexual experiences reported by female psychiatric patients. *British Journal of Psychiatry,* 160: 261–5

Parrott, L., Jacobs, G. & Roberts, D. (2008) *Stress and Resilience Factors in Parents with Mental Health Problems and Their Children.* SCIE Research Briefing 23. London: SCIE

Parsons, M. (2005) The contribution of social work to the rehabilitation of older people with dementia: values in practice. In Marshall, M. (ed.), *Perspectives on Rehabilitation and Dementia.* London: Jessica Kingsley

Parton, N. & O'Byrne, P. (2000) *Constructive Social Work: Towards a New Practice.* Basingstoke: Macmillan

Patton, G., Johnson-Sabine, E., Wook, K., Mann, A. & Wakeling, A. (1990) Abnormal eating attitudes in London schoolgirls a prospective epidemiological study: outcome at twelve months. *Psychological Medicine*, 20: 382–94

Payne, S. (1999) 'Dangerous and different': reconstructions of madness in the 1990s and the role of mental health policy. In Watson, S. & Doyle, L. (eds), *Engendering Social Policy.* Buckingham: Open University Press

Piachaud, J. (2008) Globalization, conflict and mental health. *Global Social Policy*, 8(3): 315–34

Pilgrim, D. (2009) *Key Concepts in Mental Health.* 2nd edn. London: Sage

Pinfold, V. & Corry, P. (2003a) *Under Pressure: The Impact of Caring on People Supporting Family Members or Friends with Mental Health Problems.* London: Rethink

Pinfold, V. & Corry, P. (2003b) *Who Cares?* London: Rethink

Plumb, S. (2005) The social/trauma model. In Tew, J. (ed.), *Social Perspectives in Mental Health.* London: Jessica Kingsley

Prince, M., Patel, V., Saxena, S., Mai, M., Maselko, J., Phillips, M. & Rahman, A. (2007) No health without mental health. Global Mental Health Series. *Lancet*, 370: 859–77

Prior, P. (1999) *Gender and Mental Health.* Basingstoke: Macmillan

Putnam, R. (1995) Bowling alone: America's declining social capital. *Journal of Democracy*, 6(1): 65–78

Radley, M. (2009) Understanding the social exclusion and stalled welfare of citizens with learning disabilities. *Disability and Society*, 24(4): 489–501

Ramon, S. (2005) Approaches to risk in mental health: a multi-disciplinary discourse. In Tew, J. (ed.), *Social Perspectives in Mental Health.* London: Jessica Kingsley

Rapp, C. & Wintersteen, R. (1989) The strengths model of case management: results from twelve demonstrations. *Psychosocial Rehabilitation Journal*, 13: 23–32

Raskin, J. & Lewandowski, A. (2000) The construction of disorder as a human enterprise. In Neimeyer, R. & Raskin, J. (eds), *Constructions of Disorder: Meaning-Making Frameworks for Psychotherapy.* Washington, DC: American Psychological Association

Ray, M. & Phillips, J. (2002) Older people. In Adams, R., Dominelli, L. & Payne, M. (eds), *Critical Practice in Social Work.* Basingstoke: Palgrave

Ray, M., & Pugh, R. with Roberts, D. & Beech, B. (2008) *Mental Health and Social Work.* Research Briefing. London: SCIE

Read, J. (2004) A history of madness. In Read, J., Mosher, L. & Bentall, R. (eds), *Models of Madness: Psychological, Social and Biological Approaches to Schizophrenia.* Hove: Brunner Routledge

Read, J. & Haslam, N. (2004) Public opinion: bad things happen and can drive you crazy. In Read, J., Mosher, L. & Bentall, R. (eds), *Models of Madness: Psychological, Social and Biological Approaches to Schizophrenia.* Hove: Brunner Routledge

Read, J., Mosher, L. & Bentall, R. (eds) (2004) *Models of Madness: Psychological, Social and Biological Approaches to Schizophrenia.* Hove: Brunner Routledge

Repper, J. & Perkins, R. (2003) *Social Inclusion and Recovery: A Model for Mental Health Practice.* London: Bailliere Tindall

Rethink (2006) *Sharing Mental Health Information with Carers: Pointers to Good Practice for Service Providers.* Available at www.sdo.nihr.ac.uk/files/adhoc/54-briefing-paper.pdf, accessed 5 November 2010

Rethink (2010) Government U-turn on jury service provokes urgent launch of charity campaign. Available at www.rethink.org/how_we_can_help/news_and_media/press_releases/government_uturn_on.html, accessed 16 August 2010

Ritchie, J. H., Dick, D. & Lingham, R. (1994) *The Report of the Inquiry into the Care and Treatment of Christopher Clunis*. London: Stationery Office

Rivers, I. (2001) The bullying of sexual minorities at school: its nature and long-term correlates. *Educational and Child Psychology*, 18(1): 32–46

Rivers, I. (2004) Recollections of bullying at school and their long-term implications for lesbians, gay men, and bisexuals. *Crisis: The Journal of Crisis Intervention and Suicide Prevention*, 25(4): 169–75

Roaf, C. (2002) *Co-Ordinating Services for Including Children and Young People: Joined Up Action*. Buckingham: Open University Press

Roberts, D., Bernard, M., Misca, G. & Head, E. (2008) *Experiences of Children and Young People Caring for a Parent with a Mental Health Problem*. SCIE Research Briefing 24. Available at www.scie.org.uk/publications/briefings/briefing24/index.asp, accessed 5 November 2010

Robinson, M., Atkinson, M. & Downing, D. (2008) *Supporting Theory Building in Integrated Services Research*. Slough: National Foundation for Educational Research

Rogers, A. & Pilgrim, D. (2000) *A Sociology of Mental Health and Illness*. 3rd edn. Maidenhead: Open University Press

Rogers, A. & Pilgrim, D. (2001) *Mental Health Policy in Britain*. 2nd edn. Basingstoke: Palgrave Macmillan

Rogers, A. & Pilgrim, D. (2003) *Mental Health and Inequality*. Basingstoke: Palgrave Macmillan

Rogers, C. (2003) *Client Centered Therapy*. London: Constable

Romme, M. & Escher, S. (eds) (1993) *Accepting Voices*. London: Mind

Rose, D. (2008) Madness strikes back. *Journal of Community and Applied Social Psychology*, 18: 638–44

Rose, D., Ford, R., Lindley, P. & the KCW Mental Health Monitoring Users' Group (1998) *In Our Experience*. London: Sainsbury Centre for Mental Health

Rose, N. (1985) *The Psychological Complex: Psychology, Politics and Society in England, 1869–1939*. London: Routledge & Kegan Paul

Rosenhan, L. (1973) On being sane in insane places. *Science*, 179(4070): 250–8

Roth, A. & Fonagy, P. (2004) *What Works for Whom?* 2nd edn. New York: Guilford Press

Royal College of Psychiatrists (1998) *Men Behaving Sadly*. London: Royal College of Psychiatrists

Rutherford, M. & Duggan, S. (2007) *Forensic Mental Health Services: Facts and Figures on Current Provision*. London: SCMH. Available at www.scmh.org.uk/pdfs/scmh_forensic_factfile_2007.pdf, accessed 27 January 2010

Rutter, M. (1999) Protective factors in children's responses to stress and disadvantage. In Kent, M. W. & Rolf, J. E. (eds), *Primary Prevention in Psychopathology. Vol. 3: Social Competence in Children*. Hanover, NH: University Press of New England

Rutter, M. & Smith, D. J. (1995) *Psychosocial Disorders in Young People: Time Trends and Their Causes*. Chichester: John Wiley

Sainsbury Centre for Mental Health (2002) *Breaking the Circles of Fear*. London: SCMH

Sainsbury Centre for Mental Health (2007) *Getting the Basics Right: Developing a Primary Mental Health Care System in Prisons*. London: SCMH

Sainsbury Centre for Mental Health (2008) *In the Dark: The Mental Health Implications of Imprisonment for Public Protection*. London: SCMH

Saleebey, D. (ed.) (1997) *The Strengths Perspective in Social Work Practice*. 2nd edn. New York: Longman

Samuel, M. (2009) Northern Ireland to have first unified mental health law. *Community Care*, 11 September. Available at www.communitycare.co.uk/Articles/2009/09/11/112553/northern-ireland-to-have-first-unified-mental-health-law.htm, accessed 23 August 2010

Saxena, S., Thornicroft, G., Knapp, M. & Whiteford, H. (2007) Resources for mental health: scarcity, inequity, and inefficiency. *Lancet*, 7(370): 878–89

Sayce, L. (2000) *From Psychiatric Patient to Citizen*. Basingstoke: Macmillan

Scheff, J. (1975) *Labelling Madness*. Englewood Cliffs, NJ: Prentice Hall

SCIE (2009) *Think Child, Think Parent, Think Family: A Guide to Parental Mental Health and Child Welfare*. London: SCIE

Scottish Executive (2001) *New Directions: Report on the Review of the Mental Health (Scotland) Act 1984 (Millan Report)*. Edinburgh: Scottish Executive

Scottish Executive (2007) *Effective Approaches to Risk Assesment in Social Work: An International Literature Review*. Edinburgh: Scottish Executive

Scottish Government (2009) *Towards a Mentally Flourishing Scotland: Policy and Action Plan 2009–2011*. Edinburgh: Scottish Government

Scull, A. (1977) *Decarceration: Community Treatment and the Deviant – A Radical View*. Englewood Cliffs, NJ: Prentice Hall

Seebohm, F. (1968) *Report of the Committee on Local Authority and Allied Social Services*. Cmnd. 303. London: Stationery Office

Seligman, M. (1975) *Helplessness: On Depression, Development and Death*. San Francisco: W. H. Freeman

Sewell, H. (2009) *Working with Ethnicity, Race and Culture in Mental Health*. London: Jessica Kingsley

Sheppard, M. (2002) Mental health and social justice: gender, race and psychological consequences of unfairness. *British Journal of Social Work*, 32: 779–97

Showalter, E. (1987) *The Female Malady*. London: Virago

SIGN/Mental Health Foundation (n.d.) *Executive Briefing on Mental Health Services for Deaf and Hard of Hearing People*. Available at www.mentalhealth.org.uk/our-work/all-adults/deaf-charter/?locale=en, 5 November 2010

Singleton, N., Meltzer, H. & Gatward, R. (1998) *Psychiatric Morbidity among Prisoners in England and Wales*. London: Office for National Statistics

Singleton, N., Bumpstead, R., O'Brien, M., Lee, A. & Meltzer, H. (2000) *Psychiatric Morbidity among Adults living in Private Households, 2000: Summary Report*. London: Office for National Statistics

Slater, L. (2004) *Opening Skinner's Box: Great Psychological Experiments of the 20th Century*. London: Bloomsbury

Smith, R. (2010) Social work, risk and power. *Sociological Research Online*, 15(1). Available at www.socresonline.org.uk/15/1/4.html, accessed 2 March 2010

Social Perspectives Network (n.d.) Social work identity. Extract from article in *Community Care*. Available at www.spn.org.uk/index.php?id=1090, accessed 8 April 2010

Spataro, J., Mullen, P., Burgess, P., Wells, D. & Moss, S. (2004) Impact of child sexual abuse on mental health: prospective study in males and females. *British Journal of Psychiatry*, 184: 416–21

Spitzer, R. L., Lilienfeld, S. O. & Miller, M. B. (2005) Rosenhan revisited: the scientific credibility of Lauren Slater's pseudopatient diagnosis study 1. *Journal of Nervous and Mental Disease*, 193(11): 734–9

Springer, K., Sheridan, J., Kuo, D. & Carnes, M. (2007) Long-term physical and mental health consequences of childhood physical abuse: results from a large population-based sample of men and women. *Child Abuse and Neglect*, 31(5): 517–30

Stanley, N. & Manthorpe, J. (2001) Reading mental health inquiries. *Journal of Social Work*, 1(1): 77–99

Szmukler, G. & Holloway, F. (2000) Reform of the Mental Health Act: health or safety? *British Journal of Psychiatry*, 177: 196–200

Telford, R. & Faulkner, A. (2004) Learning about service user involvement in mental health research. *Journal of Mental Health*, 13(6): 549–59

Tew, J. (ed.) (2005) *Social Perspectives in Mental Health*. London: Jessica Kingsley

Thompson, D. (2009) What does 'social capital' mean? *Australian Journal of Social Issues*, 44(2): 145–61

Thompson, N. (1995) *Theory and Practice in Health and Social Welfare*. Buckingham: Open University Press

Thompson, N. (2003) *Promoting Equality: Challenging Discrimination and Oppression*. 2nd edn. Basingstoke: Palgrave Macmillan

Thompson, N. (2006) *Anti-Discriminatory Practice*. 4th edn. Basingstoke: Palgrave Macmillan

Thompson, N. (2010) *Theorising Social Work Practice*. Basingstoke: Palgrave Macmillan

Timms, N. (1964) *Psychiatric Social Work in Great Britain (1939–1962)*. London: Routledge & Kegan Paul

TNS UK (2009) *Attitudes to Mental Illness 2009*. Research Report JN 189997. Available at www.dh.gov.uk/prod_consum_dh/groups/dh_digitalassets/documents/digitalasset/dh_100651.pdf, accessed 16 November 2010

TNS UK (2010) *Attitudes to Mental Illness 2010*. Research Report JN 207028. Available at www.its-services.org.uk/silo/files/attitudes-to-mental-illness-2010-research-report.pdf, accessed 5 November 2010

Townsend, P. & Davidson, N. (eds) (1988) *The Black Report: Inequalities in Health*. London: Penguin

Trevithick, P. (2007) *Social Work Skills: A Practice Handbook*. 2nd edn. Maidenhead: Open University Press

Trivedi. P. & Wykes, T. (2002) From passive subjects to equal partners. *British Journal of Psychiatry*, 181: 468–72

Tummey, R. & Turner, T. (2008) *Critical Issues in Mental Health*. Basingstoke: Palgrave Macmillan

Turner, O., Windfuhr, K. & Kapur, N (2007) Suicide in Deaf populations: a literature review. *Annals of General Psychiatry*, 6(26)

UNICEF (2007) *Child Poverty in Perspective: An Overview of Child Well Being in Rich Countries*. Florence: UNICEF Innocenti Research Centre

UNICEF (2008) *The State of the World's Children*. New York: UNICEF

Usher, C. (2006) Social capital and mental health in the urban south, USA: a quantitative study. In McKenzie, K. & Harpham, K. (eds), *Social Capital and Mental Health*. London: Jessica Kingsley

Ussher, J. (1991) *Women's Madness: Misogyny or Mental Illness?* Hemel Hempstead: Harvester Wheatsheaf van Ommeren, M., Saxena, S. & Saraceno, B. (2005) Mental and social health during and after acute emergencies: emerging consensus? *Bulletin of the World Health Organization*, 83(1): 1–80

Walking the Way to Health Initiative (2006) *Mental Health*. Available at www.whi.org. uk/uploads/documents/2335/Mental%20Health%20pdf%2012%20Jan%20 06%20final.pdf, accessed 13 February 2009

Wanless, D. (2004) *Securing Good Health for the Whole Population*. London: Stationery Office

Warner, R. (1994) *Recovery from Schizophrenia: Psychiatry and Political Economy*. 2nd edn. London: Routledge

Watson, S. & Hawkings, C. (2007) *Dual Diagnosis: Good Practice Handbook*. London: Turning Point

Webb, S. (2006) *Social Work in a Risk Society*. Basingstoke: Palgrave Macmillan

Webber, M. (2005) Social capital and mental health. In Tew, J. (ed.), *Social Perspectives in Mental Health*. London: Jessica Kingsley

Welsh Assembly (2005) *Raising the Standard: The Revised Adult Mental Health National Service Framework and an Action Plan for Wales*. Cardiff: Welsh Assembly

Wenger, E. (1998) *Communities of Practice*. Cambridge: Cambridge University Press

WHO (1992) *The ICD-10 Classification of Mental and Behavioural Disorders: Clinical Descriptions and Diagnostic Guidelines*. Geneva: WHO Available at www.who.int/ classifications/icd/en/bluebook.pdf, accessed 9 February 2010

WHO (2001) *Gender Disparities in Mental Health*. Geneva: WHO

WHO (2005) *Mental Health: Facing the Challenges, Building Solutions*. Report from the WHO European Ministerial Conference. Copenhagen: WHO Regional Office for Europe

WHO (2007) International Statistical Classification of Diseases and Related Health Problems: 10th revision. Available at http://apps.who.int/classifications/apps/ icd/icd10online, accessed 24 November 2010

WHO (2008) *The Global Burden of Disease: 2004 Update*. Geneva: WHO. Available at www.who.int/healthinfo/global_burden_disease/2004_report_update/en/index. html, accessed 25 August 2010

WHO (2009a) *Mental Health Fact File*. Available at www.who.int/features/factfiles/ mental_health/en/index.html, accessed 16 April 2010

WHO (2009b) *Women's Health in Prison*. Copenhagen: WHO

Wilkins, D. (2010) *Untold Problems*. London: National Mental Health Development Unit/Men's Health Forum. Available at www.menshealthforum.org.uk, accessed 5 November 2010

Wilkinson, R. & Pickett, K. (2009) *The Spirit Level: Why More Equal Societies Almost Always Do Better*. London: Allen Lane/Penguin

Williams, J. (2005) Women's mental health: taking inequality into account. In Tew, J. (ed.), *Social Perspectives in Mental Health*. London: Jessica Kingsley

Wilson, I. (2002) Case management. In Harris, N., Williams, S. & Bradshaw, T. (eds), *Psychosocial Interventions for People with Schizophrenia*. Basingstoke: Palgrave Macmillan

Wilson, M. (2009) *Delivering Race Equality in Mental Health Care: A Review*. London: National Mental Health Development Unit/Department of Health

Woodcock Ross, J., Hooper, L., Stenhouse, E. & Sheaff, R. (2008) What are child-care social workers doing in relation to infant mental health? An exploration of professional ideologies and practice preferences within an inter-agency context. *British Journal of Social Work*, 39(6): 1008–25

World Bank (1999) What Is Social Capital? *PovertyNet*. Available at www.worldbank. org/poverty/scapital/whatsc.htm, accessed 13 April 2010

Yeung, E. (2003) *Endurance: Improving Accessibility to Mental Health Services for Chinese People*. Liverpool: Merseyside Health Action Zone

Young, M. S., Harford, K., Kinder, B. & Savell, J. (2007) The relationship between childhood sexual abuse and adult mental health among undergraduates. *Journal of Interpersonal Violence*, 22(10): 1315–31

Younghusband, E. (1959) *Report of the Working Party on Social Workers*. London: Stationery Office,

Young Minds (2004) *Mental Health in Infancy*. London: Young Minds. Available at www.youngminds.org.uk, accessed 27 October 2009

Young Minds (2006) *Looking After Looked After Children: Sharing Emerging Practice*. London: Young Minds. Available at www.youngminds.org.uk, accessed 6 April 2010

Zubin, J. and Spring, B. (1977) Vulnerability: a new view on schizophrenia. *Journal of Abnormal Psychology*, 86: 103–26

STATUTORY INSTRUMENTS

The Mental Health (Approved Mental Health Professionals) (Approval) (England) Regulations 2008 No. 1206. Available at www.opsi.gov.uk/si/si2008/uksi_20081206_en_3, accessed 16 August 2010

Index

9 780745 646107